NATURAL HEALING

NATURAL HEALING
Staying Well Naturally in the Modern World

Peter Jackson-Main

AEON

First published in 2025 by
Aeon Books

Copyright © 2025 by Peter Jackson-Main

The right of Peter Jackson-Main to be identified as the author of this work has been asserted in accordance with §§ 77 and 78 of the Copyright Design and Patents Act 1988.

All rights reserved. No part of this publication may be reproduced, stored in a retrieval system, or transmitted, in any form or by any means, electronic, mechanical, photocopying, recording, or otherwise, without the prior written permission of the publisher.

British Library Cataloguing in Publication Data

A C.I.P. for this book is available from the British Library

ISBN-13: 978-1-80152-193-2

Typeset by Medlar Publishing Solutions Pvt Ltd, India

www.aeonbooks.co.uk

DEDICATION

This book is dedicated to my friends Nicolas Kinloch and Hargurchet Bhabra

CONTENTS

PREFACE
So you want to be well? ... xi
    A short personal history ... xii
    Awakening to health freedom ... xviii

CHAPTER ONE
What is Natural Healing? ... 1
    The Healing Power of Nature ... 2
    The Six Non-Naturals ... 6
    The Natural Healing Filter ... 7
    Simplicity, responsibility, change ... 10
        Simplicity ... 11
        Responsibility ... 11
        Change ... 11
    Cleansing and Rebuilding ... 12

CHAPTER TWO
Detoxification and the "evacuation of superfluities" ... 15
    Terrain over pathogen ... 17

The organs of elimination and detoxification	21
1. The bowel	22
2. The kidneys	25
3. The liver	26
4. The lymphatic system	29
5. The skin	30
6. The lungs	31
Indications for detoxification	32

CHAPTER THREE

Practical detoxification	35
The bowel cleanse	35
Bowel motility capsules	36
Drawing powder	37
Bowel cleanse diet	39
Colonics and enemas	39
The coffee enema	41
The kidney flush	42
Preparation	42
The liver flush	46
Preparation	47
Tips and cautions	49
The lymphatic system	50
Dry skin brushing	50
Hydrotherapy	50
Exercise	50
Deep breathing	50
Bodywork	50
Diet	51
Herbs	51
The skin	52
Dry skin brushing	52
Hydrotherapy	53
Topical treatments: Clay, salt and oils	55
Clothes and topical products	55
The lungs	56
Additional detox advice	56
Food intake	56
When to detoxify	57

The one-month detox programme	58
5-Day "fast-track" detox	59
Sample detox diary	62

CHAPTER FOUR
Food and drink	65
What is food?	67
Supplements	71
Optimising the fire of digestion	74
Mindful eating	76
Food combining	77
To be or not to be "Plant based"?	79
Eat the rainbow	81
Juicing	83
Cooked versus raw food	85
Water of life	86
Defensive living	87
Fasting	90

CHAPTER FIVE
Ambient air and the electromagnetic soup	93
The rabbit hole in the sky	94
Defensive strategies	98
Heavy metal detox	102
The electromagnetic soup	103
The sunshine of our lives?	106

CHAPTER SIX
Movement, rest, balance	109
Moving your body	111
The mother of yin tonics	114
Sleep hygiene	117
Dreaming	118
Awakening	119
The subtle art of doing nothing	120
Hormesis	121

CHAPTER SEVEN
Perturbations of the mind and spirit	125

Plant medicine	128
The Bach Flower Repertory	130
Physical movement	131
Bodywork	133
Purpose, and a path with heart	134
Relationships: Needing the eggs	136

CHAPTER EIGHT
Cautions, contraindications, and confidence	139
How far are you prepared to go?	140
Case 1: Iatrogenic illness: Putting your money where your mouth is	141
Case 2: Emergency medicine—a case apart?	145
Case 3: A new arrival	151

CHAPTER NINE
The spectrum of wellness	157
A bit more politics…	158
Integrated medicine	164
"A herbalist in every home; a practitioner in every community"	166
Incurable people	168
Living and dying	169
The spectrum of wellness	170

CHAPTER TEN
The space of healing	175
The critical importance of health beliefs	176
Affirmations	181
The space of healing	184
Time to heal	187
The miracle of life	188

ACKNOWLEDGMENTS	191
BIBLIOGRAPHY	193
INDEX	199

PREFACE

So you want to be well?

The primary focus of this book is to empower you to take command of your own health through natural methods. This is not a replacement for conventional medicine (until perhaps you are ready to make this transition): it is a personal practice and commitment that puts the needs of your body, which is a being of Nature, ahead of all other considerations and authorities. Once understood and adopted, the methods outlined in this book will help you to achieve lasting and powerful health, and the knowledge and skill to address problems in health as they arise.

To this end I have kept the academic paraphernalia of notes and references to a minimum and seek to speak directly to you from my own experience of what I have found to work in practice, and in recommending these methods to my clients in over forty years of professional practice as a Natural Healer and Herbalist.

My primary inspiration for this goes a long way back, but certainly major landmarks were meeting two giants of Natural Healing at a very early stage in my development. The first of these was Dr Bernard Jensen, whose influence on Natural Healing (also known as Nature Cure or Naturopathy) is legendary, and whose contribution to one of my most trusted modalities, that of Iridology, has been constitutional for that discipline. I am fortunate enough to have studied, if only very briefly, with Dr Jensen, and with others in his school and tradition, including my second major influence, Dr Richard Schulze—the "Herb Doc"—who was also a student of Jensen's.

It is to Dr Schulze that I owe some of the most cogent soundbites that act as banners in this book. For example, the three pillars of Natural Healing, "Simplicity, Responsibility and Change", which you can find (at the time of writing) reiterated on the Natural Healing page of our website. Dr Schulze, by his own admission, is a "Natural Healing Evangelist". I have constantly sought to emulate his intensely practical, but passionate "can do" approach, and in return he also graced the revised edition of my first book, *Practical Iridology*, with a glowing endorsement and foreword. I feel his influence, his love and support, every moment of my professional life.

Dr Schulze is also responsible for the critical piece of psychological software that he termed "the Natural Healing Filter", and which is discussed in Chapter 1. In an age when the word "natural" has become a passport to commercial product placement and marketing, this important "download" enables us to open up to our own intuition and inner knowing in terms of what our bodies need, and whether to trust the myriad so-called "natural" solutions out there, ever eager to promote themselves as your go-to necessities. You will learn, from that section of the book, how to deploy a few simple checks to answer any doubts you may have.

That is not even to say you may not choose something that is not strictly "natural": the key point here is that YOU CHOOSE. That is the meaning of empowerment; however, you also bear the responsibility for those choices. True Natural Healers (I should say just "Healers") do not coerce or lay down the law. They educate, they support, they counsel, they empower. They teach you to stand on your own two feet, and that is what Natural Healing has done for me. Here is a brief story of how I got started.

A short personal history

I was first introduced to Natural Healing in the late 1970s, just after I graduated from Cambridge University. I had begun my teenage years grandiosely convinced that I was some kind of magus who would be able to change the world once I had mastered the appropriate principles. I set about learning things that most teenagers never even think about—yoga, meditation, affirmation, astral travel, alchemy. I became a vegetarian, and then a vegan. I was weird. I attracted attention and puzzlement from my peers, schoolteachers, parents, siblings and pretty much everyone else unless they were as weird as me—and there weren't many of those.

I went up to University in Cambridge to study English literature in 1974, graduating in 1977. Those three years were a whirlwind of doing everything that I had been prohibited from doing while in the shelter of the family home, and not much of that was salutary, in terms of health management. I burnt the candle at both ends relentlessly, usually because I had left everything to the last minute and routinely needed to pull all-nighters to get my assignments in on time. That invariably also meant a substantial intake of caffeine, alcohol, tobacco and other substances. I sometimes did not see the light of day, especially in the winter months, getting up at 4pm or later, to pursue an alternate nocturnal career as a backgammon supremo. I was indeed well known for this, but it was not the lugubrious and relaxed backgammon of Levantine cafes and street life: it was the frenzied "win at all costs" of the dopamine addict.

While I was at university in Cambridge, UK, I registered with a local general practitioner who remains one of my biggest medical heroes and influences. When faced with the raft of random and incongruous symptoms with which I continually presented him, he would typically scratch his head, purse his mouth, and pronounce, "I have absolutely no idea what the trouble is", and then refer me to Addenbrookes Hospital for specialist investigations, which invariably turned out similarly inconclusive. But I never felt that he was failing to take me seriously; he simply didn't know and was not afraid to say so. Occasionally, if absolutely necessary (I suspect for placebo reasons rather than pharmacological), he might prescribe something anyway, but he never rushed to do so.

I loved going to see this man and was impressed by his simple honesty, which contrasted sharply with other medical people I had consulted who were over-hasty in both diagnosis and treatment. His patience and compassion were seemingly endless. Moreover, he played the cello, and so, probably over-optimistically, I regarded him as a "fellow musician", and was comforted by the notion that he had a life and purpose outside of his medical ministry, which I felt reflected balance and a sense of proportion.

Nonetheless, my health issues continued to plague me, and I them. I was, unbeknownst to my young self at that time, on a mission to dig deeper into the mystery of disease, or "dis-ease" as New Age protagonists were, even at the era, beginning to frame it. And so, when a girlfriend of mine told me of her own interest in "alternative medicine" and reported that she had found a practitioner just outside of Cambridge doing things like herbalism, reflexology and iridology, I immediately booked myself in to see her.

Her name was Farida Sharan, now well-known for her own books and teachings, and she started by looking into my eyes with a torch and magnifier and then giving me a read out of my health condition, flagging up things I had never even thought of, like bowel health, liver congestion and kidney weakness. She dispensed herbal materials into several brown paper bags and told me how to prepare them. Additionally, she told me to become vegetarian (I already was), and fast occasionally. It was she, also, at a certain point in our association, who introduced me to Dr Jensen, whom she had invited to Cambridge to conduct a week-long training seminar, to which she kindly invited me at no cost.

She also, at a certain point in my treatment, asked me, "What do you intend to do with your life?" I confessed that I had no idea. I had left university at this point and was subsisting by means of a checkered succession of temporary jobs from labouring to menial office-bound paper-pushing—or indeed, collecting social security between engagements under the dubious category of the Professional and Executive Register, which in other terms was the "dole" (social security, for those who may not know the colloquial term), but for smart kids who supposedly had prospects, except that at that era there were few prospects indeed for arts graduates outside of the university environment itself, or journalism. I couldn't stomach the thought of either and what I really wanted to do was be a musician—but I had learned that this was not something you readily admitted to unless you really enjoyed being regularly subjected to the strait-jacketing opinions of those who believed it "impossible to make a living" that way. Farida suggested I fill in time by taking some of her natural healing classes, to which I enthusiastically agreed.

And thus, my career was initiated, in the curious way that life has of guiding you to where you are supposed to be, almost accidentally, or by default. I took the herbal medicines, and the dietary suggestions, and I did the "cleanses" with alacrity, which was like being scoured from the insides out; and I felt almost immediately better for it all—three or four years of stagnation and rust pretty much gone in a few weeks.

In quick succession I then covered anatomy and physiology, massage, aromatherapy, reflexology, and then Polarity Therapy. The latter was the subject that really grabbed my attention, mainly due to its strongly eclectic theoretical foundations that called on everything from Taoism and Ayurveda, the Hermetic tradition, quantum physics and contemporary cosmology. But beyond its arcane epistemological foundations I discovered a resolutely "hands-on", practical, experiential system of holistic health care whose relevance to the modern world and its dilemmas could scarcely be denied. Very simply, I was hooked—on the gift of Natural Healing, the endowment of the vital universal energy upon each of us, which uniquely bestows the power to address any imbalance, any assault, any error, any injury.

I was fortunate indeed to discover this all well before reaching the age of thirty. I remember this often when consulting with clients who are significantly older, sometimes several decades older, and who have had the time to accumulate the ravages, not only of time and an often less than salutary physical and social milieu, but of the orthodox system of health management itself, with its "no going back" surgical interventions, and its toxic chemicals masquerading as medicines.

Even so I had myself lost organs, before all this was revealed to me— the ones you can "do without", obviously (how many of those are there, I wonder?). The tonsils and adenoids went at age six, the appendix at age eleven. It would be disingenuous of me to claim, with respect to the latter, that the intervention was malign or ignorant since I would undoubtedly have died from peritonitis if not for the surgery and antibiotics. Surgery has been practised by humans for at least two thousand years, and I am quite certain that if antibiotics had been around two thousand years ago, we would have been using them too. In a way we were, of course, since herbs have long fulfilled the need for antisepsis in medicine and are still pretty good at it today.

So often, however, it is our own situation that guides us to the work we need to be doing, and such was the case with me. In those days there were no stand-alone courses in the UK teaching what I wanted to learn, so I set out to learn everything possible by means of short courses and of course seeing as many practitioners as a patient as I could possibly find—or afford.

It was through my attendance at one of these clinics, at a certain point in my approximately 15-year-long extended training period, that I eventually came upon Dr Christopher's School of Natural Healing.

Dr John Raymond Christopher was the legendary North American Eclectic herbalist who specialised in treating cases of near-impossible severity with herbs and Natural Healing. I had been introduced to his work by the first practitioner that I ever saw, straight out of university in the 1970s, so it seemed auspicious that this tradition had once again presented itself to me.

I was especially impressed that his school, and his book of the same name, used the term "Natural Healing", as opposed to "The School of Herbology" or "The School of Herbal Medicine". Again, there were other schools operating in the UK that taught herbal medicine, and I could have studied with any of them, but I was looking for something very specific. Having already met Dr Bernard Jensen and been awe-struck by his encyclopaedic knowledge and his eclectic naturopathic approach, I quickly realised that this was the tradition in which I would be most at home, and the unifying factor was that the teacher on this course, Dr Schulze, had been trained by both these two giants of Natural Healing: this was the biggest attraction, and the cause of considerable excitement not only for myself, but for others in my circle. I had already studied anatomy and physiology along with my massage and aromatherapy training, so I was able to go straight into Herbal Medicine.

Once I had made the decision and committed to it, things moved fast to enable my next step, which was to enrol in the next cohort, the first session of which was to take place at a retreat in southern Spain in the autumn of that year, which was 1992. The course fee was way beyond my means, but very quickly and entirely unexpectedly I was presented with a bursary from a hitherto unsuspected source, which enabled me to pay for the course.[1] I just had to find the air fare.

There followed modules in natural nutrition, iridology, detoxification, hydrotherapy, bodywork (including more Polarity Therapy), and clinical internships. This school was resolutely practical, so all teaching was embedded into personal lifestyle and habit, and became the bedrock of an already well-developed understanding of the precepts of Natural Healing, turning me out onto the streets in 1994 as a fully-fledged Natural Healing Herbalist. My life partner and closest friend and ally, Anji, also registered on these courses and graduated a year later, so together we set up The Natural Centre for Herbal Medicine, Iridology and Natural Healing, and opened ourselves to receive enquiries.

We were still grindingly poor at the time, having now spent all our money on training (and having a young family as well), and I remember phoning Anji one evening from Spain and saying, "Clean out the outhouse for when I get home: we're opening a herbal dispensary!" On my return we did just that, but with no money to afford stock, we bought just one litre of tincture of hawthorn berry. It amuses me now to think of the faces of some of my more conventional colleagues in the profession when I report that our first few patients therefore all got a prescription of hawthorn, no matter what they presented with. Of course, they also got a ton of natural healing advice on diet and lifestyle! In a short space of time, we had enough money to replace the hawthorn and buy a second litre, this time of cramp bark, and so on and on until our shelves were eventually fully stocked with a comprehensive range of herbal medicinal extracts.

I am immensely proud of the way in which we accomplished our success, even before we found the School of Natural Healing, applying the principles we had already gathered in our journey so far, working through thick and thin (mainly thin), step by step, inch by inch, to establish ourselves doing exactly what we wanted to do, in the face of a good deal of ignorance, and some fairly unpleasant exchanges with "colleagues" who did not approve of our training (while of course knowing nothing about it) because it was not *their* training. Anji, who also had a passion for animals, particularly dogs, had also familiarised me with the work of Juliette de Baïracli Levy—her own legendary heroine of natural healing. Juliette's classic, *The Natural Rearing of Children and Animals*, had been Anji's go-to resource for Natural Healing since long before even we met.

In all of it we resolutely stuck to our principles of Natural Healing— our diet, lifestyle choices, medical choices, and the raising of our three (later four) children was resolutely "natural", sometimes to the point of obstinacy, but it paid off: our children, although we were poor, were never sick, never in the GP's surgery, let alone the hospital. In the first year of our partnership we lived (by chance and necessity) in an old farmhouse, run as a communal house. It was freezing in the winter and there was no central heating, while in the summer it was fly-ridden and right next door to a cesspit. The cats, dogs, goats and chickens, who were also our co-residents, were far less problematic than the people: the social aspect of it was everything you were always warned about in terms of communal living: contentious, brittle, squalid, and completely devoid of appropriate boundaries.

Into this situation our third child (actually Anji's third, my first) was born, to the absolute horror of the attending midwife, after a completely natural and uncomplicated pregnancy, on a mattress on the floor of our one room. The joy and the sheer vibrant vitality of the occasion was the only infection to which we fell prey. Shortly after that, and probably because the "authorities" were eventually persuaded that the situation was not suitable for the raising of very young children, we were offered council accommodation—a three-bedroomed semi-detached property on the outskirts of Cambridge, with a large garden. This was the home of the first incarnation of The Natural Centre, and we ran a practice from that address for the best part of a decade.

The rest, as they say, is history—or at least a story for another occasion—but the reason for sharing these details with the reader here is to try and bust another popular contemporary myth: that natural living is expensive and privileged. IT IS NOT. The means and the methods described in this book are within the reach of most people who have a little space to call their own; and the knowledge to begin making the relevant choices is accessible to all.

Above all, as will become obvious, Natural Healing is a mindset, a philosophy if you like, but a coherent world view or metaphysics. In addition to the practical wisdom it encompasses, in terms of physical healing, the *attitudes* of "Simplicity, Responsibility and Change" are in themselves profoundly transformational, and can function tacitly to overcome the obstacles that we can often put in our own paths, in terms of unhelpful beliefs and habits of thought. Sometimes the trappings and comforts of contemporary living can work in the opposite fashion, to reinforce those beliefs and habits, taking us further away from what is really important in our lives. We did not exactly *enjoy* being poor, but it focused us very differently, and in many ways it was a healthy existence, free of distractions and superfluities, closer to the earth and to the seasons and cycles of the planet, closer to our authentic selves, perhaps.

Awakening to health freedom

My experience in Dr Schulze's class did one other thing for me. It brought into full and powerful focus that committing to Natural Healing, herbal medicine and a diet of natural and organic foods is truly an act of resistance. I remember writing at one point in some correspondence I was conducting, that I believed medicine to be, as-yet unrecognised, the most important political issue on our planet. I do not mean the "philanthropic" initiatives to make pharmaceutical medicines and vaccinations available to children in Third World countries. I do not even mean the pioneering policy of Aneuran Bevan in mid-twentieth-century Britain founding the National Health Service, healthcare "free at the point of delivery"—although I do support that initiative.

What I mean is something far more radical. In citing an "act of resistance" it becomes necessary to define exactly what we are resisting. In my mind this came to its fullest expression yet in the circumstances of the global SARS-Cov-19 pandemic of 2020 and the events that followed. I was deplatformed three times for advising people to use natural methods to stay well during this time, and for amplifying the notion of natural human immunity developed and maintained by such practices. It was clear to many of us during that time that the major threat we were facing was not the virus, but something far worse and more insidious: that the pandemic was being used to roll out a blanket global treatment and containment strategy that admitted no competitors; and all of this was accomplished by engineering abject terror into a defenceless population. And when fear of "the virus" started to wane, or be subjected to questions, it was transferred on to fear of the loss of our liberty: take the offered medical solution OR …. Lose your freedom, lose your job, find yourself unable to move freely around the planet, be unwelcome in the social space, suffer reduced access to services including food and routine medical assistance; but perhaps most frighteningly, suffer reduced access to EACH OTHER.

Whatever your personal reaction or response to these events was—whether or not you chose to bow to the pressure to receive the offered medications, whether or not you chose to comply with lockdown, mask-wearing or social distancing—freedom was forfeit for all of us. Not just the freedom to move around, either locally or globally but, implicitly, the fundamental freedom to choose what we may or may not put inside our own bodies. In the UK clever language was used to the effect that, while it was never actually illegal to pursue an individually determined path through this event, most people thought that this was the case and complied with the "mandates" on that understanding, while those who didn't were vilified and ostracised.

For me it was very clear from the start how this would play out. On day one I predicted the fast-tracking of a vaccine within the year, and a global mandate to take it or be left out of society. Nonetheless

I knew that I would never willingly comply with this. My faith in my own immunity after decades of natural living was absolute, and my fear of the vaccine was always more vivid than any apprehension I may have had about the "virus".

Subsequent to the acute events, of course, the woefully inadequate clinical trials, the raft of serious, life-threatening "side-effects", the mysterious "excess deaths situation" that received hardly any coverage in the mainstream media, the admissions by senior medical advisors such as Anthony Fauci that mask-wearing was never going to protect anyone from anything and could possibly exacerbate respiratory distress, and the high probability that the "virus" itself was a bioweapon released from a laboratory facility working (apparently) on devising novel ways to kill people, have all become common knowledge to anyone who has kept even half an eye on developments. Those of us condemned as "conspiracy theorists" and socially irresponsible purveyors of misinformation have been vindicated many times over as the truth leaked, almost unobtrusively, into the public domain.

In short, there has never been a better time to promote natural healing, and natural *living*, as a viable alternative to remaining at the mercy of a monolithic medical system that has proudly proclaimed the creation of no fewer than nine new billionaires within the pharmaceutical industry alone, as a direct result of the pandemic, and on the back of widespread human suffering.

Many found themselves looking for a better way, and those of us who had been lucky enough in life to have already found this were suddenly busier than we had ever known ourselves to be in the service of educating, promoting and informing our fellow citizens in the ways of natural living and strategies of both prevention and cure.

The result is that many have discovered that the "side effects" of this approach to personal healthcare—enhanced immunity, vitality, longevity and effective self-regulation—deliver far more than they had ever thought possible, used as they were to being fully reliant upon standard, conventional health care; and as the National Health Service in the UK continues to be dismantled and sold off to corporate interests around the world (who clearly have no real interest in maintaining the health of people who are not even near-neighbours, let alone fellow country-men and—women and co-citizens), the knowledge of how to preserve and maintain personal health on a day-by-day basis, and how to harvest the cumulative benefits of natural living, is precious indeed.

So, if for you, as for me, health is freedom, the freedom to create abundant vitality and joy in your lives and those of your close companions in life; if you aspire to be free of the sometimes depressing predictions and prognoses of standard medicine, and the lifelong prescriptions of drugs with all their side-effects; if you, like me, believe in the awesome power of Nature to address the severest and most intransigent of "diseases", then this book may be for you. You will not, however, find full "scientific" validation for every statement that I make; you will not get statistical facts and figures until they fall out of your ears; you will not get formulaic responses to each and every disease and "condition" that you might experience along your life path.

What you will get, however, is foundational. You will learn how to live naturally in the service of both prevention and cure. You will learn how to regulate and govern your own energy and vitality. You will learn simple routines and ideas by which to accomplish correct nourishment, detoxification, relaxation, recreation and regeneration. You will learn the theory and the practice of self-regulated natural health care.

So: you want to be well? Let's begin!

Endnote

1. In this I remain to this day indebted to the offices of Rhea Monroe, who facilitated this financial intervention. I cannot even recall the name of the Foundation from which the funds were made available, but I can only hope I have fulfilled my part of the bargain, which was to use the knowledge for the healing and education of as many people as possible. This book is part of that unwritten contract.

CHAPTER ONE

What is Natural Healing?

Natural Healing, also known as Naturopathy, or Nature Cure, is a healing philosophy and practice that is based upon the idea that Nature is the only and the ultimate source of all healing, and that healing itself depends upon promoting, unblocking and harmonising the body's own natural vital energy. It is an extremely ancient practice that can be traced back through the aeons to the remotest periods of human civilisation and beyond. It is implicit in the precepts and philosophies of the great sage, Hermes Trismegistus (also known as Thoth in the Ancient Egyptian tradition);[1] in the mythological pronouncements of the Greek demigod Asclepius and his daughter Hygieia; and in *The Essene Gospel of Peace* discovered and translated from the Aramaic by the Hungarian philologist Edmond Bordeaux Szekely in the 1920s,[2] purportedly relating to the original teachings of Jesus two thousand years ago.

I choose the term Natural Healing over Naturopathy simply because I was trained in Dr John Christopher's "School of Natural Healing". Christopher was a surviving member of the Eclectic medical movement in North America, which was almost entirely dismantled in Abraham Flexner's Rockefeller-funded reforms of medical schools in 1910. As one of America's foremost proponents of herbal medicine, I have always regarded it as highly significant that he chose to call both his school and his seminal book, not the *School of Herbology*, or the *School of Herbal Healing*, but the *School of Natural Healing*. The significance is that even while using herbs as his foremost healing modality, his overarching rationale for using them, along with his dietary strategy and other healing practices, owed itself to a fundamental belief in the healing power of nature itself.

The Healing Power of Nature

The single most important thing to understand about Natural Healing is that the clue is in the name: the healing is *always* done by Nature. This includes healing that takes place in the context of standard medicine, in hospitals, under the knife, and in the presence of consumed pharmaceuticals.

Sometimes we might be tempted to say, *in spite of* these conditions, since in strict naturopathic terms most of these interventions are suppressive: they are predicated upon the removal of the symptom—whether the literal removal of tissue that is presumed "diseased", or the removal—or masking—of a symptom that the body has created either with the intention of righting a wrong (vomiting, for example, to get rid of noxious material in the stomach), or to bring the problem to the conscious awareness of the individual—pain of any kind has this function.

The body always acts to survive and redress, although too often we see these efforts as evidence of disease—we frequently confuse the symptom with the disease. Books with titles such as *The Healing Power of Illness*,[3] and *Love Your Disease, it's Keeping you Healthy*,[4] suggest that we become familiar with the idea that the way illness and disease is framed in the contemporary world is mistaken, or just plain wrong. Less than a hundred years ago in 1932, American physiologist Walter B. Cannon published *The Wisdom of the Body*.[5] Bearing the subtitle, *How the human body reacts to disturbances and danger and maintains the stability essential to life*, the book is possibly the first comprehensive exposition of the scientific concept of homeostasis, and makes a very similar point, framing illness as a corrective phenomenon, aimed at restoring homeostatic balance.

The concept of the Healing Power of Nature is a very old one, and it is echoed in ancient humoral medicine systems from around the world where they have survived. In the European humoral medicine tradition, it is sometimes referred to using the Latin phrase, *Vis Medicatrix Naturae*—of which it is a literal translation. It is closely allied to the concept of *Energetics* (for a discussion of this term see Chapter 1 of my previous book, *The Mind's Eye*[6]), for it assumes that at a fundamental level everything is *energy*.

This is not so far removed from some of the tenets of contemporary science that we cannot fathom it and connect it to everyday experience. We know that matter is only "solid" in our perception of it. In the ancient systems of healing this "power" had a few different names: the Greeks called it *pneuma*, and connected it with breathing and the lungs; in the Indian tradition it is *prana*, and again linked to breathing and air (the practice of *pranayama* in yoga is a breath practice); and in traditional Chinese medicine it is called qi (pronounced 'chee')—and *everything* is qi, ultimately. Qi that can be used by our bodies is also partly formed in the lungs from the qi in the air.

In contemporary terms we might also invoke the concepts of *non-locality* and *entanglement* to illustrate the way this might work: non-local effects are those that are faster than the speed of light, in other words do not conform to the usual limitations of time and space. Entanglement, technically, describes the natural connections that apply within a multipartite system represented by a single quantum state. Again, this can take place across time and space, and the concept has been used to explain the healing action of homeopathic remedies.[7] When healers talk about "healing energy", for example, they often observe that this can be directed across distances, and both backward and forward in time.

In terms of our bodies, whether or not you are prepared to admit to believing in some arcane supernatural power residing "in the air", you will still be familiar with the concept that when injured, the body will attempt to heal itself: the scientific physiological concepts of inflammation and homeostasis, properly studied, cannot fail to lead to the conclusion that biological systems are equipped *by Nature* to self-repair and self-regulate. The only argument—a metaphysical one with which we do not have to engage fully here—is where the energy comes from that performs these "miracles".

The point is, you do not have simply to *believe* in the Healing Power of Nature: you can see it in action every day in your own body. When you cut yourself do you not heal? When you become ill with an infection does the body not usually deal with the infection and return itself to health? (Or is that just the paracetamol and/or antibiotics?) Does not your body manage itself continually to maintain a correct tissue environment through the operation of homeostasis?

A brief look at what is known as the "natural history of inflammation" will reveal the truth of these matters. When you cut yourself there is first bleeding, redness and pain. The bleeding stops at a certain point, but the redness continues. This redness is evidence that the process of inflammation is now at work: the blood vessels in the area have become porous to allow immune cells to move into the surrounding tissues to begin the clean-up process. When that is done, the blood transports nutrients to the area to start the rebuilding and remodelling process. Eventually, when everything is done, there is a perfect repair, without a scar. Scar tissue is evidence that some "filler" has had to be used—not always a bad thing, but suggesting that for whatever reason, the job could not be completed as a "perfect" repair—usually due to a shortfall of nutrients, to the presence of foreign material that could not be removed, or to the failure to immobilise the injury site.

So, the body has done what it needs to do to ensure the ongoing functionality of the organism. The time it takes is commensurate with the depth and extent of the injury. To be sure, we assist in this consciously through the administering of hygiene techniques, ambulatory support, and bone-setting, for example, but the actual *healing* is accomplished by Nature, according to the inherent physiological programming with which the body is endowed.

This is a description of *acute* inflammation: but what of *chronic* inflammation? Is this not evidence of the body somehow misjudging the matter and keeping the inflammation going long after it should have been turned off? A quick trawl of the internet will indeed bring up a hundred examples of the prevailing narrative: "acute inflammation = good; chronic inflammation = bad". Certainly, chronic inflammation can be painful and destructive, but let's look a little closer.

In the process of researching this phenomenon I consulted the evidence base through my favourite search engine, Ecosia. They had recently installed an AI function to answer questions, so I overcame my natural resistance to AI and decided to consult the database of knowledge to which the AI clearly had easy access.

At first, I got the standard answers, for example, "Autoimmune conditions like rheumatoid arthritis or lupus involve the immune system mistakenly attacking healthy tissue." I did not settle for this, and I commented: "The idea of immunity 'mistakenly attacking healthy tissues' is an example of an interpretation of the phenomenon of chronic inflammation, and not necessarily a true one."

Ecosia replied, "You are correct that the concept of the immune system mistakenly attacking healthy tissues in autoimmune conditions is an interpretation of the phenomenon of chronic inflammation and not an absolute truth," but still reiterated: "It is essential to recognize that the immune system's response can sometimes be misdirected or overactive, leading to chronic inflammation and associated health issues."

Again, not satisfied, I submitted the rejoinder: "Suppose that the body has not switched off the inflammation because it knows that the underlying problem has not been dealt with: what evidence is there to show that the 'triggers' of chronic inflammation may be the problem here, and not the 'immune dysregulation' that is assumed?"

Ecosia replied: "Research suggests that chronic inflammation can indeed be triggered and perpetuated by ongoing factors such as infections, environmental toxins, dietary choices, stress, and lifestyle habits, among others. Addressing the underlying triggers is crucial in managing and reducing inflammation levels. By identifying and addressing these triggers, such as adopting a healthier diet, reducing exposure to environmental pollutants, managing stress effectively, and making lifestyle changes, it is possible to help the body switch off chronic inflammation and promote overall well-being."

Now compare this list of healthy habits with The Six Non-Naturals (below), and you will clearly see that contemporary "Artificial Intelligence" has eventually been persuaded to validate the Natural Healing approach. Note especially the phrase, "… to *help the body* switch off chronic inflammation" (my italics). I am beginning to appreciate the possible advantages of an impartial logical intelligence over the programmed bigotry of human scientists with an agenda!

The natural conclusion here is, if your body is producing a "symptom", it probably has good reason to do so. The underlying triggers, whether those are to be found in retained environmental toxins, or in the concept of "stress"—that little word that covers such a multitude of ills—are what we should always be looking for. The ongoing inflammation is a critical signal that indeed all is not well, and that we should continue to look for, and address, the root of the problem.

Indeed, we could say that an indwelling intelligence, hardwired into the intimate physiology of our systems and constantly working on our behalf—an intelligence that will not be satisfied with incomplete answers and botched attempts to suppress natural reactivity—is a highly likely hypothesis, based on the available evidence.

However, as always, it is completely up to you whether or not to accept this hypothesis in full. All we need for now is that you are prepared to consider that the body, being a *natural* phenomenon, is capable of healing itself, and in fact strives to do so at every opportunity. This means that even things that hurt—illness and pain—have a purpose and may be regarded as the clues we need to follow in order to discover the reason for, and relieve ourselves of, the problem.

The next step is the realisation that "natural" is not something external to us; it is not a mere marketing tag added to foods, supplements, household cleaning products, textiles and so on, to convince us that the seller has our interests at heart and that we are somehow safe to buy these things. Natural is not a commodity. Natural is a state of being, and one from which we cannot escape. Natural will always follow certain laws, the laws of the natural world, certainly, but we ourselves are part of the natural world. We arose out of it, and eventually we will capitulate to it. In the meantime, the strong suggestion implicit in the pages of this book is that, for best results in healing, we are best advised to live closely within those laws.

The Six Non-Naturals

This is where the "non-naturals" come in. The Six Non-Naturals is a concept from the ancient medicine of Europe, thought to originate with the Roman physician Claudius Galenus—commonly known as Galen[8], and also found in Middle Eastern "Tibb" medicine. But why "non-naturals"? Simply, because these are not innate as such: we can choose. We can choose to live in a fashion that ignores the laws of Nature; or we can choose to live close to those laws. It is up to you what food you put in your mouth, whether to exercise, sleep, or indeed maintain the equilibrium of your mind or the cleanliness of your bowels.

The list of the Six Non-Naturals is as follows:

- Ambient air
- Food and drink
- Exercise and rest
- Sleep and wakefulness
- Elimination and retention
- Perturbations of the mind and spirit

These factors at one and the same time signal the importance not only of the issues we need to address in order to heal—and to remain healthy—but also point towards the confounding factors that undermine health, the *allostatic load*, which is the sum of all the environmental influences, physiological, psychological, emotional and energetic toxins, against which homeostasis has to struggle in order to maintain viability.

Since knowing what to do about all these factors forms a major part of the advice given in a Natural Healing context, a full discussion of each of the Non-Naturals will be given in subsequent chapters, and some attempt will be made to disentangle and resolve the heady complexity of competing do's and don'ts. First, however, we will need to install a piece of psychic software called the "natural healing filter" to enable the reader to see through the plethora of obfuscations to divine for herself the truth in any situation.

But the overarching message is, YOU CAN MAKE A DIFFERENCE. *You can help your body to heal itself,* through the everyday choices that you make.

The Natural Healing Filter

In an age where information and disinformation coexist in every area of life, where black is declared white and truth falsehood, it is necessary to have some means of deciding for ourselves that which we can trust and rely on. Nowhere is this more necessary than in the attainment of health and the management of disease. Science says, "Trust me!", but then spoils itself by remaining resolutely impregnable to alternate perspectives and new information. The glass ceiling operates to refuse entry to those who do not recite the accepted canon, and the tag "pseudoscience" or even "conspiracy theorist" is liberally slapped on those who are determined to stick their heads above the parapet and challenge the accepted view of things. I have personally been "cancelled" and deplatformed several times for attempting to repeat this advice on social media.

And so, I pass on to you the download that I received more than thirty years ago while (literally) sitting at the feet of Dr Richard Schulze: *The Natural Healing Filter*. This critical discriminatory tool will assist you to make decisions in relation to your health challenges according to what is likely to help, and what to hinder your progress. It is not the ultimate authority on everything. It is still open to you to make either informed or intuitive choices to use other methods as appropriate to your situation.

In practice I use this method as a guide to answering certain questions that I am routinely asked, particularly about whether my patients should use such and such a product, or nutritional supplement (nutraceutical). Quite frequently, when I recommend a herb instead of a supplement, the question comes back, "Which brand should I buy?" I might say, "Nature's Own", but then I am drawn into explaining that I just made it up to make a point, so now I say, "Go down the road, take a right, then a left, then you'll see a field in front of you: THAT brand!"

I have never forgotten the following story, relayed to us in herbal class by the Herb Doc himself.

The renowned Dr Christopher was once invited to speak at a trade fair of purveyors of various herbal and nutritional products. I have attended and exhibited at many such events myself, and the array of products, panaceas and potions is truly bewildering. Sitting in our booth with our humble cellophane packs of dried organic herbal teas, and brown glass bottles full of traditionally produced extracts, we often felt very much like the poor relation beside the glittering array of blister packs, cleverly chelated mineral solutions and arcane electronic wizardry—all purporting to be "natural".

Christopher spent the first hour or so of his visit pacing up and down the aisles looking at the products on display, and then finally arrived on stage to address the expectant multitudes, overlooking the arena with all the stalls and pop-up shops. He began, "Well you know, I've walked up and down these aisles and looked at all your attractively packaged supplements, and I have this to say. There is one problem with all of it." At this point he banged his fist down on the table in front of him and thundered, "They're all DEAD!"

Amid the pandemonium that ensued the celebrated doctor was swiftly ushered off the dais and out of the hall.

Schulze's own view, promulgated in the classroom, reinforces the point: "I see my patients coming in with armfuls of these products that they are taking, but when I ask whether they are feeling better from them, they say no. They pee orange but they don't get better."

Do not misunderstand, I am not here to tell you not to take your supplements if you are convinced about them, but my own experience is very similar to the two doctors'. In some cases, I have seen people spending up to four hundred pounds a month on supplements, which are clearly not working, because otherwise why would they be in my office? They have come with the expectation that I am going to give them another supplement that is going to be the clincher. Then they ask me which of the thirty-odd products that they have emptied onto my desk they should continue to take, and which they should not. I have two possible reactions to this—one is to be "reasonable" and subject each offering to the appropriate scrutiny, but in doing so to lose the will to live; the other is to advise them to dump the whole lot into the trash and start over.

If, like me, you are convinced by the Healing Power of Nature, and you want to make that a leading principle in your health choices, then this range of questions is designed to bring you to the understandings that you need to make your choices:

1. How close is this product to the way that Nature originally intended it? If a herb, for example, what care has been taken to preserve its unique original properties? Traditional preparation and storage methods have proven reliable over millennia to preserve the medicinal virtues of herbs: is this product truly an improvement on those, and if so, how?
2. How much processing has this product been subjected to, and what materials have been used in the processing? Chemical solvents, for example, are frequently used in advanced extraction methods: to what extent might this be an adulterant in the finished product?
3. How much energy and money in terms of advertising and marketing has been put into promoting this product? Products placed on social media, for example, often come with promotional videos that can take up to an hour to view, while piling on the pressure to buy with the frequent appearance of "click bait". This is high-pressure selling and is driven by money, not by a healing initiative.
4. What is the nature of the science that supports this product, and how has it been conducted? There are few things more obfuscatory than claims of "scientific" veracity: frequently they rely on the purchaser knowing little or nothing about "the science" and being hypnotised into accepting the tag "science" or "scientific" as a badge of quality and reliability.
5. Has animal testing been used in the development of this product? In the herbal profession in the UK, for example, there is an implicit understanding that these methods are not appropriate in a natural healing context. Apart from the ethical issues and the

very real possibility of animal cruelty, the science behind animal experimentation is dubious in its transferability to humans.
6. What is the *philosophy* behind the product? This in my view is the most important question. Does this product truly support the assumption of a natural healing force (the Healing Power of Nature), or is it based on an atomistic notion of purely chemical effects? Is it in any meaningful sense ALIVE? Or is it, as Dr Christopher pronounced at the trade fair, DEAD?
7. Lastly, why do I NEED this product? Is it because I have been TOLD I need it? Is there another way in which the same benefit might be gained, but in a less expensive or more holistic manner? For example, could I get this nutrient by eating FOOD, as opposed to taking a supplement?

Simplicity, responsibility, change

Here is another great formulation that once again I owe to Dr Schulze. These three principles are foundational in the philosophy and psychology of Natural Healing. Together they supplement the Natural Healing Filter by providing a template for personal engagement with the inherent healing capacity of our own bodies and minds.

We can frame and discuss them in relation to three Great Myths of Healing that apply in our time. These myths are built into the very fabric of our thinking in terms of healing, until we learn to recognise them, deconstruct them and put something better in their place. It goes like this:

Myth One: "Diseases are complex and various, and the ways to conquer them are also therefore complex and various."

Actually, the causes of all diseases are remarkably similar and simple, and so are their cures.

Myth Two: "Illness is a misfortune that strikes from outside ourselves."

Actually, most illness arises from inside you, and is often Nature's way to guide you to take command of your own life.

Myth Three: "To get well I need someone clever to do something clever (that I don't understand) to me."

Actually, you can heal yourself. You just need to change the way you think and act in relation to your own health.

Simplicity

In Naturopathic theory and philosophy we find the idea of the "Unity of Disease", which is the idea that "illness" is predicated upon a very simple understanding of the way that tissues and organs become deranged. For example, we can take the energetic theory of the blockage of vital energy being the source of imbalance. Or we could focus on the notion of toxic encumbrance of the tissues, causing injury and inflammation, which is also connected with the idea of acid–alkaline balance (see Chapter 2). In scientific terms this is not so far removed from the idea of homeostasis, the natural balancing act performed by the body to keep everything in a state of healthy functioning.

Responsibility

From there we go on to discover what it is that is causing that blockage, and our own role in maintaining the perceived distortions, whether that be by our lifestyle, our diet, or our very thoughts. No matter that we may feel that someone or something else has been instrumental in injuring us and "causing" our disease, no one ever got well by complaining about it. Even if you think it wasn't your "fault", once you have found the cause, it is completely up to you to take responsibility for how you now address it going forward. It's all very well to blame your situation on something external, but then to carry on expecting that something external is going to be the answer makes little sense. Learn the lesson!

Change

The courage and the commitment to make the required adjustments is the natural follow-through. It has been said that to carry on doing the same things while expecting a different result is a true definition of stupidity. We are all prone to stupidity from time to time, but in the service of reclaiming our health, it is a luxury we can ill afford (pun intended). No one said change is going to be easy, but having dealt with the two principles above, we at least now know what needs to be done. It is now down to us, and us alone, to make the changes required, and commit to them.

Cleansing and Rebuilding

The final baseline principles of Natural Healing that I wish to present to the reader are the twin pillars of Cleansing and Rebuilding. The practical detail of these principles follows in Chapters 2, 3 and 4, but it is worth introducing the concepts as foundational to Natural Healing.

A builder does not take on a plot and just start erecting new structures upon it. There is a need to clear away the rubble and debris of what was there before. Even if it had not been previously built upon, there will be a need to remove the undergrowth, to level the land, and create a firm foundation for the new structure. There will be a need to ensure that there is nothing in the terrain that will cause problems later down the line—toxic deposits, sink holes and subsidence, or the presence of certain plants that are able to break up concrete and destroy buildings.

Similarly with the body: clean, positive health cannot be built upon a filthy terrain (see Chapter 2 for a brief discussion of Terrain Theory). This was probably the very first lesson in my own studies in Natural Healing, and we were taught simple and immediately effective methods of performing the appropriate cleansing and preparation. This is clearly about "detoxification", which can be a more in-depth process, according to individual need and history, and this in-depth discussion will be the subject of the next two chapters.

Building health is then predicated upon doing things differently from that moment onward—building, indeed, healthy practices and habits instead of reinforcing the old unhealthy ones. This is where we engage with the basic principles of Natural Living and strive as far as possible to integrate them into our lives as securely and comprehensively as possible. This enhanced Natural Healing practice forms the majority of the material that follows in this book.

One final word, and a caveat, about these principles: nothing replaces the need for individual, personalised advice, especially in the case of chronic or seemingly "complex" pathology. In professional naturopathic practice a guiding principle would always be the individual diagnostic information gathered during the course of a proper professional consultation. In fact, treating the person, not the disease, and treating the whole picture, not just the symptom, are both vital principles in Natural Healing practice. <u>If in doubt, always consult a qualified, registered natural health professional.</u>

Endnotes

1. Lachman, G. (2011). *The Quest for Hermes Trismegistus* (Edinburgh: Floris Books).
2. The Wikipedia entry on *The Essene Gospel of Peace* states that these four documents are now regarded as forgeries, but there are clear resonances with material found in the Dead Sea Scrolls and the Nag Hammadi texts from Egypt.
3. Thorwald, D. & Dahlke, R. (1995). *The Healing Power of Illness* (London: Element).
4. Harrison, J. (2018). *Love Your Disease: It's Keeping You Healthy* (London: Atlantic).
5. Cannon, W. (1963). *The Wisdom of the Body*. New York: W. W. Norton and Company Inc. Cannon's book also highlighted the physiology of the "stress response", and arguably prefigured the work of Hungarian-Canadian endocrinologist Hans Selye in his book *The Stress of Life* (1956), which relates to material to be discussed in Chapters 6 and 7 of the present volume.
6. Jackson-Main, P. (2024). *The Mind's Eye: Personality and Behaviour as Revealed in Quantum Iris Analysis* (London: Aeon).
7. Milgrom, L. (2008). A New Geometrical Description of Entanglement and the Curative Homeopathic Process. *Journal of Alternative and Complementary Medicine*, 14(3): 329–339.
8. It has been pointed out that the expression is not found in the writings of Galen, but is more probably an articulation of Enlightenment physicians. See Jarcho, S. (1970). Galen's Six Non-naturals: A Bibliographic Note and Translation. *Bulletin of the History of Medicine*, 44(4): 372–377. http://www.jstor.org/stable/44450783.

CHAPTER TWO

Detoxification and the "evacuation of superfluities"

A ccording to contemporary nutritional theory, detoxification is no longer a thing. It has been debunked, disproved, is no longer valid, no one needs to bother about it any more. Traditional naturopaths can all pack up and go home.

The trouble with pronouncements like this is that they are generally made by people who have never done a single day's detoxing in their lives. If they had they would have some personal experience to add into their theoretical bombast. But no, we must believe "the science", and the science says that it's hooey, bunkum, hogwash: *pseudoscience*, indeed.

Several years ago, I was watching the ITN lunchtime news on 2 January, and they ran a semi-serious magazine feature (after all the reports on war and murder, human tragedy at the hands of natural disasters, the interest rate hikes, the nefarious international political shenanigans) on the quaint little custom of January detox. They lined up four experts—three doctors and a nutritionist—and they posed the question, "why detox?"

So, 2 January is the day AFTER the monumental national hangover: having "celebrated" not just at Christmas, but in an escalating three- or four-week preparatory run-up to the grand event, the good people of our land, after a period of intermittent torpor in the week after

Christmas, top the whole cocktail off with a humongous festival of self-harm known traditionally as "New Year's Eve".

Starting a brand-new year off by being ill has never really been attractive to me, so of all the nights I generally choose to be at home in front of the fire, this is the "no-brainer". (I'm being slightly mischievous of course ... I've done my fair share of partying, for sure—that's how I know!) But for many of our number it is the occasion of another popular tradition, the New Year's Resolution, and in a desperate attempt to reverse the damage, on waking to the cold light of day people resort to all kinds of equivocations with their gods—and their bodies—to commit to more constructive lifestyle practices. Small wonder, really, that 2 January is the most popular day to "throw a sicky". (All that detoxing takes planning and attention to detail!).

So, the question first went to two of the doctors: "Why detox? Is it necessary?"

"Well, no not really. Your body is fully equipped to do its own detoxing, there's nothing you can do to speed that up. All you need to do is eat healthy, drink plenty of water, ensure restful sleep, and you'll be fine."

Coming to the nutritionist, the same question: "I really have nothing to add to that: healthy food, plenty of water, plenty of rest, that's the recipe."

The third doctor was obviously a cut above the rest, because they left him till last. He was from Cambridge (my home city) and was obviously cleverer; and he said, "Yes, all of the above ... It does help to have a good liver though!"

My first—sarcastic—response was, "OK let's go down to the butcher's shop and get one, shall we?" But then I thought, has this man just accidentally (or cleverly) shot the entire argument down? If we accept that liver function has a role to play in detoxification (something of a no-brainer there, I think) then we should be asking the question, "Is there something we can do to enhance or optimise liver function?" If nutritionists are saying "no", then they need to explain why many of their number are routinely prescribing milk thistle, or glutathione, or NAC (n-acetyl cysteine)? Not to mention optimising diet by ensuring plentiful amounts of antioxidant-rich foods and the specific nutrients that support liver detoxification pathways?

You cannot have it both ways. Either natural therapies work, or they don't. If you shoot down detoxification, you need to be very careful that you are not just cravenly playing into the hands of the "scientific" cartels that would like people to believe that none of these practices have any validity.

But the real message here does not depend on any theoretical discussion: it is squarely based on actual practical experience. This is the only way you will learn if detoxification protocols "work", or not. Your barometer is <u>how you actually feel</u> for having done them, not what some superannuated professor is telling you to believe.

In the herbal medicine degree-level diploma course that I administer, we have an assignment near the beginning of the period of study that requires students to perform, on themselves, a simple detoxification routine. They choose between protocols addressing the bowel, the kidneys, the liver, and the lymph, and they explain the reasons for their choice by reference to their own health patterns, and then plot their progress on a daily chart, measuring such criteria as energy levels, hunger patterns, frequency of bowel motions, and other symptoms such as headaches and digestive discomfort, or any persistent problem that they may be dealing with.

The assignments thus produced make for eye-opening reading. The simplest routine that they may choose is arguably the Kidney Flush (see Chapter 3), and many choose this for reasons of simplicity and time-management. Even the simple practice of drinking lemon juice in water in the morning, with the addition of a few drops of extract of cayenne pepper, produces results that astonish the students themselves, and is a solid testimony to what can be achieved with an absolute minimum of effort.

So do not lecture me on the redundancy of detoxification until you have done at least one of these routines and observed and experienced their effects for yourself.

Terrain over pathogen

The significance of Terrain Theory is discussed in the 2023 edition of my book, *Practical Iridology*.[1] Briefly, for these pages, at the turn of the nineteenth and early twentieth centuries two competing paradigms battled it out for supremacy in medical science, the second being Germ Theory. Germ theory held that disease was caused by the damage inflicted on tissues by microorganisms. Louis Pasteur (of pasteurisation fame) and his close associate Robert Koch (discoverer of the tuberculosis bacillus) were successful in establishing Germ Theory as the prevailing medical model, over the efforts of Pierre Antoine Béchamp and Claude Bernard (the originator of the term "terrain" in a medical context, and arguably the forerunner of the later concept of homeostasis), who declared that the microbe was of no consequence in a clean and healthy terrain. Béchamp even went so far as to aver that microbes as such arose not externally but were innate in the body and came with the purpose of scavenging tissue that had become diseased through disturbance of the terrain.[2]

Even Rudolph Virchow, one of the most important influences on standard modern medicine, owing to his discovery of cellular pathology as the basis of disease, reportedly declared towards the end of his life that if he had his time over, he'd spend it proving that diseased tissue was the preferred habitat of "infective" organisms, rather than a consequence of them.

Terrain theory predicts that the susceptibility or vulnerability of the organism to immune challenges and supposed external threats is a function of the viability and the vitality of its organs and tissues. In contemporary biomedical terms we have a concept that is similar if not identical—that of *homeostasis*. Homeostasis is the complex set of operations that maintains the optimal temperature, pressure, pH, hydration and nutritional status that our physiology needs for correct functioning. Injury, whether by means of physical trauma, extremes of temperature, depleted nutrition, chemical and biological toxins, or radiation, will temporarily or permanently undermine the balance of homeostasis, either locally or globally, and calls forth a healing mechanism called *inflammation* in order to return the organism to functional normality. As we have seen, among inflammation-prolonging influences we find heavy metals, chemical and biological toxins, and nutrient depletion, but also key disturbances of terrain, such as hypoxia and acidosis, which are in fact related.

An example of how we think about this can be seen in the naturopathic theory concerning pH balance (acidity vs alkalinity). The ideal pH for human blood is between 7.35 and 7.45 on a 15-point scale—in other words, pretty much bang in the middle, neutral. Too far outside either of these parameters will seriously undermine health. pH is closely allied to oxygen provision: when blood pH is unbalanced, as in acidosis, then hypoxia ensues—and hypoxia itself is another example of the "Unity of Disease" discussed in Chapter 1. Nobel Prize-winning scientist Otto Warburg's theory that cancer thrives in the context of an anaerobic (oxygen-depleted) metabolism has theoretically never been overturned, no matter that the current trend in medicine is still to dismiss it.

Therapies and nutritional programmes that correct pH and strive to improve the provision of oxygen to all cells and tissues are an important focus within Natural Medicine, and you can find detailed instructions in my first book, *Practical Iridology*, under the section on the Hyperacidic Diathesis. Another useful tool in this is the "Acid–Alkaline Food Chart", which is reproduced here. The ideal ratio of foods that cause acidic residues versus those that result in alkaline residues is 20/80 in favour of the latter. Note that this is not a comment on whether or not the foodstuff *contains* organic acids; lemons, for example, contain citric acid but do not *cause* acidosis—indeed they are part of the cure for that situation.

Food type	*Acid-forming*	*Alkaline-forming*
Beverages	Alcohol, coffee, black tea, sugary drinks, fruit juices. Rice, oat and soy milks are mildly acidic.	High pH water (8 or above), green drinks, almond milk, coconut milk.
Animal foods	All meats, shellfish, farmed and ocean fish, eggs, dairy produce. Wild freshwater fish is only mildly acidic.	None.
Grains	Most except quinoa and buckwheat.	Quinoa, buckwheat, spelt.
Pulses	Black beans, chick peas, kidney beans.	Lentils, tofu, butter beans, soy beans, white haricot, sprouted pulses.
Nuts & seeds	Brazil, pecan, hazel, sunflower.	Almonds, chia, flax seeds, coconut.
Fruits	Dried fruit, apple, apricot, peach, banana, grapes, mango, orange, pineapple, strawberry, berries.	Lemon, lime, avocado, tomato, grapefruit.
Vegetables	Mushrooms, potatoes (except new baby potatoes).	Most, including all leafy greens, carrot, broccoli, brussels sprouts, cauliflower, asparagus, artichoke, onion, red onion, zucchini, rhubarb, peas, swede, turnip, parsnip, new baby potatoes.
Other	Sunflower oil, grapeseed oil, artificial sweeteners and flavourings.	Most herbs and spices; avocado, olive, coconut & flax oils. natural salt.

Figure 1. The Acid/Alkaline food chart.

In terms of Natural Healing we will also need to factor in the sufficiency of "life energy" (prana, qi, pneuma, the Healing Power of Nature): this at the present era is unquantifiable in terms of conventional externally derived investigative methods—tests, scans, X-rays etc.—but just because science cannot find it does not mean that it is not there. Traditional medicine diagnostic techniques such as tongue and pulse analysis provide cogent methods by which this vitality may be apprehended and assessed in its physical manifestation in any person at any particular moment in time. However, it is also the case that all the injurious factors mentioned above will, if we do not manage them appropriately, deplete vitality, chiefly in calling continuously upon the inner resources of the organism in relation to the need for inflammatory—or corrective—response.

Detoxification alone will not address all the needs that this situation calls for, but it will be a vital first step. The "evacuation of superfluities", as the ninth-century Arab physician Ibn Bhutlan colourfully phrased it, is of course one of the six non-naturals discussed previously (elimination and retention) and is critical in more ways than one.

Firstly, it is necessary to remove disease-causing residues. These, by the way, are not exclusively derived from our environment. Many are created "in-house" by our own metabolic processes. Metabolism may be described as the sum of all anabolic (building, nourishing) and catabolic (detoxifying, eliminating) processes. In point of fact, these are inextricable one from another. The process of eating, for example, generates nutritional energy, but it also generates toxins—waste products—that must be eliminated (some more quickly than others) efficiently. The waste generated by the digestive process is significantly more harmful if that process is itself inefficient or lacking in vitality. Thus, traditional medicine diagnostic formulations explain that the shortfall in digestive power itself creates toxic build-up—in the Ayurvedic tradition, for example, low Agni (fire of digestion) gives rise to Ama (disease-forming substance—see Chapter 4).

Thus years, possibly decades, not only of poor food choices, but of suboptimal digestive function, may result in a significant build-up of such materials, which, by definition, are undermining health, by causing a situation again known in traditional medicine as *stagnation*. I personally prefer the term "tissue encumbrance", to describe the accumulation of metabolic wastes that have overwhelmed the organism's ability to correctly process or to eliminate—and that is before even we start talking about the additional burden of environmental toxins, heavy metals, and so-called "forever chemicals", about which we will have much to say in due course.

Terrain-modulation is nominally a complex issue, but in fact, practically speaking, its various parameters will be quickly brought into balance as soon as the impediments to the free circulation of vital energy are cleared. Whether you want to talk in simple terms of optimising the eliminative organs to do their job, or whether you want to get involved in discussions of enzyme activity and pH balance, the actual methods by which these effects are accomplished are similar if not identical.

One of the reasons I am so enamoured of plant medicine is because the medicine of plants is so multifaceted: a herb that "dredges" the liver is frequently also a herb that acts to enhance bile production (thus also working against constipation and retention in the bowel), to enhance digestion (thus reducing the accumulation of toxic and acidic accumulations), to balance the microbiome of the gut (thus reducing the likelihood of leaky gut syndrome and autointoxication), and to activate the pancreas (thus improving digestion and sugar balance, and normalising the appetite in the direction of healthier foods).

Chapter 3 gives the methods of natural detoxification and explains how the various protocols work to accomplish the desired aim of removing stagnation and relieving tissue encumbrance, thus facilitating the free flow of vital energy throughout the system. Before we get there we need to ensure we understand what is involved, and in what order to do things.

The organs of elimination and detoxification

The key organs and systems that need to be addressed in a detoxification programme are as follows:

1. The bowel
2. The kidneys
3. The liver
4. The lymphatic system
5. The skin
6. The lungs

Although some talk of a "correct" order of procedure in addressing these organs, it can be a highly individual matter. For example, if the bowel is assessed as working more or less correctly, but the liver is assessed as being stagnant and congested, the practitioner might decide to address the liver as a priority. In any case, liver therapies can often have a knock-on effect of speeding up or enhancing bowel function—there is more than one way to address any diagnosed shortfall.

Nevertheless, for the purposes of simplicity the above order of procedure is recommended. I will firstly look at the role of each of these organs, explain its place in the sequence and examine the wider impact of the organ upon other organs and systems, and the organism in general. Then, in Chapter 3, I will give the specific protocols for addressing each stage of the detoxification process.

1. The bowel

A congested bowel puts pressure on the rest of the system through autointoxication. Autointoxication means that toxic material retained in the bowel finds its way back into the blood stream, and must therefore be reprocessed by liver, kidney and lymph. In iridology, the presence of "straw yellow" cloudy appearances in the iris suggests that retained acidic material may be putting pressure on the kidneys as organs of elimination, resulting in tissue encumbrance and acidosis.

The products of liver detoxification follow two routes out of the liver: one is via the "antiporters" across the hepatocyte cell membranes into the biliary tract in the form of bile, which acts as a digestive fluid, but which is also an effluent, enabling the products of detoxification to pass out of the system with the faeces; the other is passed into the blood stream and transported down to the kidneys for filtration and elimination.

In the first case, we have the added complication that liver detoxification processes may actually be undone if conditions are not ideal in the bowel. In the case of female reproductive issues due to oestrogen dominance, for example, excess oestrogen is "conjugated" in the liver, which means that it is bound up with molecules that render it inert as it exits the liver. Passing into the bowel via the biliary tract, it may then meet a specific enzyme (beta-glucuronidase), which acts to split up the conjugated molecule, freeing up the oestrogen, which is then reabsorbed into the blood stream to further exacerbate the problem. The solution is to establish correct speed of bowel transit, as also to provide additional binding through appropriate intake of fibre, which has the function of binding toxins for safe and efficient release—belt and braces!

In terms of the lymph system, 50% of this crucial system of drainage and circulation of immune capacity is located around the gastrointestinal tract in the form of the GALT—gut-associated lymphatic tissues. This tissue maintains immune surveillance for the gastrointestinal system, but also acts as a collection reservoir for waste materials, which are then drained into the colon for elimination. Thus, the lymph system, which has no discreet outlet to the external environment, discharges via the gastrointestinal tract, and also via the blood stream (to be filtered by liver and kidneys).

Lastly the lungs. It may not appear obvious how clearing the bowel potentiates the lungs, but in naturopathic terms we recognise an innate sympathy between mucous membranes wherever in the body they occur, such that by addressing the mucosa of the gut we also reflexologically affect mucosa in other systems—respiratory, urinary and reproductive.

In Traditional Chinese Medicine, particularly, there exists a specific affiliation between the lungs and the colon. The truth of this was not lost on TCM doctors treating the initial outbreak of Covid-19 in Wuhan at the very start of the pandemic. They found that the "cold damp pestilence" affecting the lungs of Covid patients could in some cases be eased and dispersed by ensuring correct evacuation of the bowels. It is a trick that I myself used to excellent effect in treating Covid and Long Covid in the UK during the ensuing months and years of the pandemic.

Dr Bernard Jensen is probably the most prolific exponent of the fundamental importance of bowel cleansing in health maintenance, prevention and cure, so much so that he wrote a book with one of the most functional titles out there in health terms: *Tissue Cleansing Through Bowel Management* bears testimony to the primary role of correct bowel function in detoxification, and the profound impact this has on the organism as a whole.

Jensen also gives us a chart of bowel reflex connections to other organs in the body. If you look at the way that the organ reflex zones are arranged around the central portion of the iris in Iridology, which is the stomach and intestinal reflex area, Jensen suggests that each portion of the bowel is reflexologically connected to the organs immediately adjacent in the iris chart Figure 2. Sometimes there needs to be a slight stretch of the imagination to grasp this, but in other instances it is immediately obvious.

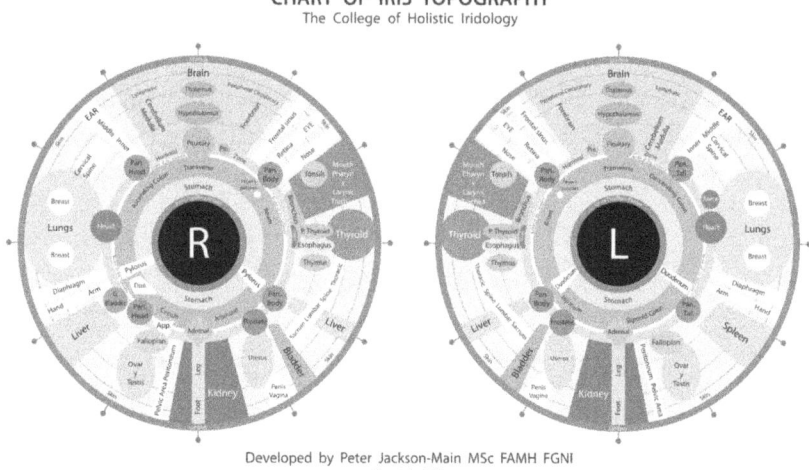

Figure 2. Chart of Iris topography.

For example, both the caecum (bottom right section of the colon) and the sigmoid (bottom left) are anatomically in close proximity to the ovaries, such that we could say that congestion, dysbiosis (imbalance of gut flora) and inflammation may exert a directly adverse influence on those structures. Moreover, the sigmoid colon wraps itself around the back of the uterus. In cases of disease of the female reproductive tract, then, the cleansing of the bowel is a fundamental necessity. I have seen dysmenorrhoea disappear almost instantly, ovarian cysts reduce in a few months, and successful implantation occur in a few weeks after months or even years of unsuccessful attempts at conception, following just one application of the bowel cleanse protocol.

Cleansing and optimising the bowel, as many naturopaths will confirm, is the first and most important stage in a detoxification programme, and it lays the foundation for addressing each of the other organs in turn. As so often in these endeavours, it is to the plant kingdom that we will turn for the most effective answers in promoting healthy bowel function.

We cannot leave discussion of the bowels without reference to desired frequency of motions. There are radically differing ideas here, with some doctors reassuring their patient that whatever is normal for them is "normal". When asking patients about their bowel habits one of the most frequent responses is, "Normal". What colour are your stools? "Normal". What consistency? "Normal". Others know that they "should" be having at least one motion daily, and some are familiar with the Bristol Stool Chart, which depicts a range of appearances, from constipated, through "normal" and healthy, to loose stool and diarrhoea, designed to deliver more precise information—it's a handy tool in consultation.

My own belief, based not purely upon precept and theory, but upon personal experience, is that the optimal frequency is one motion for each meal that we eat, and approximately 20–30 minutes after each meal. In scientific terms, this is a mechanism called the *gastrocolic reflex*, which acts to signal the colon to produce a peristaltic contraction in response to every meal. Some people are worried that this means that transit will be too quick … I then explain that it's not the SAME food coming through that you have just eaten! But if you think about it, it makes sense. Why store it all up for one release per day, per two days, per week, etc., when you may be able to achieve a uniform flow—one batch in, one batch out? It's something to aim for, but it may not be easy. There are many things that may need to be adjusted—including emotional and psychological taboos—in the quest for the perfect motion! But when you achieve it, even if only temporarily, you will know that it just feels right.

2. The kidneys

The idea behind the order of detoxification is that we prepare organs and systems that are required to handle waste by ensuring that the exit channels are clear and optimised in advance. Hence bowel first, and then kidneys and bladder, as these are the main exit channels.

We may regard the kidneys as fundamentally important from an energetic point of view also, in their reality as the "seat of our vitality"—a function that sits most comfortably in the category reserved for the adrenals in Western terms. But it is to their filtration and elimination functions that we look to them in this context. A major consideration is that, as mentioned above, some of the products of liver detoxification are shunted down to the kidneys for elimination. Therefore, kidney support may be regarded as a baseline for liver detoxification, alongside the bowel, of course, so it makes sense to ensure the health and efficiency of the kidneys and the bladder—the urinary system—

before promoting liver detoxification. Therefore, the kidneys are second in order of detoxification.

Conventional physiology has it that kidney cells, once destroyed do not regenerate. This is in stark contrast to liver cells, which are replaced in full every six weeks. Liver cells are exposed to huge amounts of oxidative stress as a result of chemical detoxification processes, and the need to constantly replace them is paramount—you have probably heard of the herb milk thistle, which has a role to play in both protecting and promoting the replacement of liver cells.

The orthodox view of the kidney, however, is that its cells are not capable of regeneration once destroyed, and thus once we have lost kidney function we never get it back. Whether or not you are disposed to believe this (they once said neurons, including those in the brain, could not repair or replace themselves: we now know that is not true), it does make sense to service and protect the kidneys on a regular basis. The kidneys also have many other interactions within the body, having a role to play, for example, in maintaining blood pressure, pH balance, fluid balance, the production of red blood cells and the maintenance of healthy bones.

There are many herbs that can contribute to the healthy function of the kidneys, not just the diuretics, which activate and promote urination, but strengthening, cleansing and nourishing these all-important organs. We will meet some of these plants in the practical advice in Chapter 3 below.

3. The liver

When people talk of "going on a detox", they frequently think of the liver as the main focus of this activity. As we have already seen, however, the liver in turn is reliant on other organs of elimination to perform its functions of neutralising and eliminating waste products and toxins.

The liver is the chief chemical factory within the body, synthesising and storing vital nutrients, monitoring and protecting against the influx of foreign materials entering the body (including food, drink, medicines and drugs), neutralizing and eliminating what is either potentially harmful or ingested in excess of natural needs, and in addition providing invaluable support to the digestive system.

So why third in line for detoxification? Well, as already explained, the liver does not have a direct exit channel to the outside world. It relies on the bowel and the kidney to handle the effluent that it produces.

Optimising bowel and kidney therefore can be said to "take the pressure off" the liver by providing an easy and efficient means of finally eliminating the products of detoxification and preventing them from being recycled and having to be detoxified all over again ... and again, and again. Reabsorption of toxins from the bowel and/or the kidney back into the blood, and therefore back though the liver, is possible, not to say likely, when these organs themselves have not been correctly managed.

The purpose of liver detoxification is to render "xenotoxins" (toxins entering the system from outside) water soluble for excretion though the kidneys. It is variously described as having between two and five "phases". I generally teach three main phases, as follows:

Phase 1 consists of enzyme activity focused primarily on "priming" toxins for conjugation (see Phase 2). The specific enzymes here are given the scientific name of "the CYP450 isoenzyme supergene family". They prime a binding site on the toxin that enables it to be "conjugated" with a suitable molecule that renders it, temporarily at least, inert and safe. However, while it is waiting for the correct molecule to be provided, it is temporarily even more dangerous than it was originally. We'll refer to this later.

There are over 50 different CYP enzymes, each suited to a specific type of toxin, and each given a numeric nomenclature that identifies the "pathway" through which specific toxins must pass in order to be detoxified. For example, pharmaceutical medicines frequently use a pathway called "CYP3A4". It is also the case that certain foods, and especially herbal medicines, may modulate these pathways in either upward (inducing) or downward (inhibiting) ways. This is why herbal practitioners working with patients on pharmaceutical medications have to know which herbs might interact with these substances.

Phase 2 is the location where the primed toxins meet their partners for conjugation. Whereas phase 1 renders toxins temporarily more toxic, conjugation in phase 2 makes them inert and safe. Once again, different species of toxins require different partners, and there are six different pathways here, each providing specific chemical substances needed for the detoxification to be completed. These substances all come from the foods we eat (or we can choose to take supplements to provide them) and may therefore be in short supply if diet is not optimal. Most of them are to be found in a variety of fruits and vegetables, and this is the single most important reason why a high intake of such foods is considered essential for optimal health.

This is partly why, when we get to the chapter on food, we will be emphasising fruits and vegetables as primary and fundamental in a health-supporting diet. We can all remember having been told, for example, that eating broccoli is not just "good for us", but also protects against many chronic degenerative diseases, including cancer, which is principally owing to the fact that the sulphur compounds in the cabbage family at large are specifically required by certain liver detox pathways, thus enabling the liver to protect the system from the possibility of harm ensuing from rampant free-radical damage caused by unconjugated toxins.

The problem with a typical contemporary diet is that these nutrients may be significantly lacking, and therefore liver detoxification may be impaired—in other words, there is a high demand for detoxification, owing to the widespread availability and incidence of environmental toxins, but often a restricted ability to respond with appropriate chemical binding.

Phase 1, typically, is activated by any number of routinely encountered toxins, not just the individually chosen habits of alcohol and tobacco consumption and poor-quality foods, but also a chemically contaminated water supply, toxins in foods arising from the almost universal use of agrochemicals, and a very high incidence, at the time of writing, of airborne toxins. If Phase 2 is impaired, nutritionally speaking, then these very dangerous substances, made "temporarily" more dangerous by the CYP enzyme activity, build up in the liver and may cause extensive damage. A sign that this is happening is the phenomenon of "liver stagnation", which may be diagnosed by traditional means, as well as from typical conditions and symptoms, way before it eventually manifests as an abnormal blood test in the form of raised liver enzymes.

Liver congestion (stagnation) may be suggested in a variety of common complaints, including headache, migraine, eye and ear problems (including tinnitus), skin outbreaks, immune problems, menstrual problems, even musculoskeletal problems, and disturbed blood sugar, to name but a few. The various parameters of liver stagnation reach into almost every area of our Natural Healing enquiry—for example, even the ability to detoxify from airborne pollutants rests finally with the optimum functioning of this organ. Remember, ANYTHING that gets into the blood eventually goes through the liver. The liver IS therefore frequently the chief target of "detox" routines, although, as we have seen, priming the bowel and kidney in advance can significantly impact upon the success and completeness of liver detoxification protocols.

Phase 3, sometimes not mentioned in physiological accounts (or seen as part of phase 2), is also known as the "antiporter" phase. Antiporters are chemical and ionic species that assist with the transport of water-soluble conjugated toxins across the hepatocyte (liver cell) membranes and into the biliary system as components of bile, whereby they are enabled, as previously discussed, to exit the system via the digestive tract. The importance of understanding this is that in detoxification we frequently use plant medicines that have the specific function of promoting bile production and secretion.

These plants, frequently known as "bitter tonics" for their ability to improve digestion, are also often the "liver dredgers", part of the "alterative" category in herbal medicine, which means they purify and cleanse the blood stream. Not all alteratives work the same way—some address kidney function, some activate the lymph system—but many act on the various phases and pathways of liver detoxification. We will be meeting some of them in the practical section on liver detoxification, in chapter three.

4. The lymphatic system

The lymphatic system may be defined both as the body's main drainage network, and a vital means of circulating immune capacity. The lymphatic circulatory channels form a parallel circulatory system to the cardiovascular system, except they do not have the heart to pump the fluids through them. I will refer to this again in chapter three in talking of the methods of priming and activating lymph flow in a detoxification programme.

Lymph is pervasive throughout the body via vascular channels that pick up and recycle wastes and circulate immune capacity to deal with any threats that this material might be found to contain. At intervals along lymphatic vessels we find "lymph nodes"—bundles of tissue that serve to filter and cleanse the circulating lymph, for which purpose they are supplied with large quantities of white blood cells, especially macrophages (literally "big eaters"), which will work to neutralise invading threats, or pathogens, and absorb and break down foreign material.

As already mentioned, the lymph system itself has no direct external outlet: it relies on discharging firstly into the blood stream for onward transit to liver and kidneys, or into the bowel, specifically the large intestine. That is the reason why there is little point in inducing or increasing lymphatic activity until those channels have been addressed and optimised. Otherwise, the material will just keep on circulating and recirculating. It is always better to unblock the drain, rather than to hand-bale the basin!

Moving lymph, however, is a necessary part of maintaining health. As mentioned, lymph does not have a central pump, like the heart for the cardiovascular system—although we could say that the operation of the thoracic duct, the central lymph channel, when correctly activated by means of exercise and deep breathing (see below) performs a similar function. But it would still be correct to state that lymph only moves if you do, and so we will see the importance of physical exercise in the maintenance of lymphatic health, as well of course as the plants that can assist.

5. The skin

In placing the skin fifth, I intend neither to downgrade nor de-emphasise its importance. In point of fact, we could say the care of the skin, for its own very individual function, should be an ongoing concern in a health-conscious lifestyle. The skin is your barrier and your boundary, but is a porous boundary and, when functioning correctly, will enable you to both excrete and ingest according to need and desire.

In terms of elimination and detoxification it is perspiration that defines the function of skin, and in health this organ (arguably the largest organ of the body) will eliminate about 2–4 litres daily through perspiration. In this capacity it has also been found to be protective to the kidneys, especially when those organs may be damaged or compromised: "the potential of urea excretion via profuse sweating is apparent particularly when the kidneys are damaged or their function is impaired".[3]

It is for this reason that, although I have placed the skin in fifth position, I will most frequently advise my patients to begin skin-enhancing practices such as dry skin brushing, magnesium or Dead Sea salts baths, and topical hydrotherapy, from the outset of a healing and detoxifying programme.

Finally, we should again mention the power of herbs to promote elimination through the skin. These plants are known as *diaphoretics* in herbal medicine, and there are basically two types—the heating and the cooling. Heating, or stimulating, diaphoretics include pungent herbs such as cayenne pepper, garlic and ginger, and they work by driving the "heat" (toxins) from the core towards the periphery for discharge via sweating. They are most useful in cases where congestion has become chronic—this may be regarded as the definition of stagnation, which tends to settle in the internal organs and need activating—heating and mobilising—in order to be released.

The second type of diaphoretic is the cooling, or relaxing, variety, including herbs such as peppermint, elder and yarrow. These work by relaxing the nerve supply to the skin pores, allowing them to open up and release sweat. This type is most useful in cases of fever, when heat is building up within the body and needs to be released in order to cool the system. The combination of herbs mentioned above is one of my favourite ways to treat colds and 'flu, where, by aiding the discharge of sweat, they enhance the action of the immune system in its attempt to address a homeostatic imbalance.

6. The lungs

The final exit channel that we need to briefly discuss is the lungs. We have already mentioned that general detoxification, especially through the bowel, can greatly reduce the pressure on these organs, which are arguably the most important organs of ingestion that we have. As Dr Schulze frequently reminded us in herbal class, "You can go a few weeks without food; a few days without water; but without oxygen you'd last only minutes."

In the chapter below on "Ambient Air" (one of the six non-naturals, if you remember from Chapter 1), I will be discussing a development across our entire world whereby air quality is being compromised in a way that is increasingly difficult to escape from. The task of cleansing and strengthening our lungs is one of the most serious measures in protecting ourselves from the adverse impact of these practices. I am talking about high-altitude chemical spraying conducted in the service of weather control and "solar radiation management". In my practice I have seen a huge upsurge of respiratory complaints presenting in my patients—phlegm that they cannot get off their chests, coughs that won't go away for weeks. At first, I thought it was the impact of Covid-19, but then I began to notice, in myself as well as my patients, patterns of respiratory distress that directly coincided with periods of fully obvious and visible high-intensity aerial activity.

We will be talking about ways of combating this in Chapter 5. For now let's just note that the necessity to address the lungs specifically as part of a detox routine has never been more pressing.

Indications for detoxification

The accompanying chart can be used to identify the need to detox. Although I recommend detoxification as routine health maintenance for everyone, if you have an existing condition that you are working with then detoxification can also be targeted to your specific condition, and although the full detox catalogue can be deployed in any situation, for each condition there may be one or two organs or systems that should be prioritised. The chart can guide you to the ones you need to focus on in particular.

For these purposes I have restricted the specific channels to the main four—bowel, kidney, liver and lymph. Best is to service each of these regularly, but you can also choose to focus on specifics. You will see that the more serious and chronic the problem is, the more channels potentially need to be addressed. If an organ is not highlighted against a specific problem, this does not necessarily mean it is not important to consider. Individual presentation is always the best guide to what needs doing in any case.

Indication	Bowel	Kidney	Liver	Lymph
Frequent infections			x	x
Fatigue—post-viral or chronic	x	x	x	x
Skin complaints	x		x	x
Headaches	x		x	
Sleep disturbances			x	
Digestive problems	x		x	
Constipation	x		x	
Obesity	x	x	x	x
Arthritis and rheumatism	x	x	x	x
High blood pressure		x	x	
Water retention		x		x
Diabetes	x	x	x	
Cancer	x	x	x	x
Cardiovascular disease	x	x	x	
Autoimmune disease	x	x	x	x
Allergy	x		x	x

Figure 3. Indications for detoxification.

Endnotes

1. Jackson-Main, P. (2023). *Practical Iridology* (London: Aeon).
2. Béchamp's final publication, The Blood and its Third Element, expounds the theory of pleomorphism, which describes the ability of microbes to change form in response to environmental cues. This phenomenon is now increasingly recognised in microbiology. See for example Doolittle, W.F. (2013). Microbial Neopleomorphism. Biology & Philosophy, 28: 351–378. https://doi.org/10.1007/s10539-012-9358-7.
3. Huang, C. et al. (2002). Uric Acid and Urea in Human Sweat. *The Chinese Journal of Physiology*, 45(3): 109–115. Available at: https://www.researchgate.net/publication/10698087_Uric_acid_and_urea_in_human_sweat.

CHAPTER THREE

Practical detoxification

In this chapter I will outline the practical methods of addressing each of the above-discussed channels, and then wrap them all into a one-month programme that I use with most, if not all, of my clients at this time. We will begin with the bowel.

The bowel cleanse

The bowel cleanse is based on herbal formulae devised by Dr Richard Schulze and Dr John Christopher, and used in deep tissue cleanse routines on patients with serious chronic disease. It is therefore a powerful cleansing routine with significant health benefits and can be used by all as a preventive measure to keep the bowels clean and free from obstruction. It should be performed over two or three weeks, at a frequency of approximately once per year—except in more serious conditions, when it may be repeated at six-monthly intervals.

Please note, however, that it is better to perform this routine for the first time under the guidance of a qualified practitioner who is specifically trained and experienced in this protocol.

There are two basic herbal formulae required for this programme: the bowel motility capsules, and the drawing powder.

Bowel motility capsules

These contain herbs that have strong laxative effects, alongside herbs that help to tone the gastrointestinal mucosa, as well as having antiseptic and balancing effects on the microbiome, discouraging and down-regulating pathogenic species while simultaneously promoting beneficial species.

I work with two strengths of these agents, which I call Intestinal Formulae (IF) 1, and 3 (IF2 is discussed below). The precise instruction is that if you are currently experiencing fewer than one bowel motion daily, you should begin by taking one of these formulae before committing to the IF2 powder, and preferably the stronger formula, in order to establish a healthier frequency.

Intestinal Formula 1: This is a very strong laxative formula originally devised by Dr Schulze, containing the most powerful anthraquinone-containing herbs to be found in the plant world. Anthraquinone glycosides exert a laxative effect by stimulating the peristaltic motion of the gastrointestinal smooth muscles and are found in large quantities in aloe species plants, as well as senna (leaf or pod) and cascara sagrada bark. These herbs are combined with pungent and stimulating herbs, cayenne, ginger and garlic, and barberry bark—itself a great gastrointestinal antiseptic and terrain-managing herb.

For those who are experiencing at least one bowel motion per day, the Intestinal Formula 3 is the usual option. For these people the number 1 capsules are too strong and will result in the necessity to be only a few steps away from the toilet at all times during the cleanse, which is neither ideal nor necessary for the success of the programme.

In fact, I once ran a herb class in the north of England among students many of whom had been seeing a particular practitioner in that area. They reported to me how fantastic the bowel cleanses they had done with this practitioner were. Intrigued, I asked for more details. I was told, you take one of these capsules with each meal, which gives you about 6 to 10 bowel motions daily. Asking about the consistency of motions, as I suspected, these were loose and explosive—and rather uncomfortable, as I also managed to get them to admit. However, when I asked them, "What about the powder?", they simply looked blank. "Did he not give you a drawing powder to absorb the toxins and the waste material and help to evacuate them?"

He did not, it turned out. Instead, his patients were given the IF1 formula, which induced diarrhoea for two weeks, under the sadly mistaken impression that they were cleansing their bowels. That is not a bowel cleanse: that is laxative abuse.

The IF1 capsules are for those with significantly less than one motion daily. If in doubt about this, I find in the UK most people are fine with the IF3 capsules, which you can easily take more of if one per dose does not work. Schulze devised the IF1 for the kind of presentation he was routinely encountering in the USA—people who might, if they are lucky, have one bowel motion per week—or who, on occasion, were not having bowel motions at all, but using colonics instead.

The IF3 capsules contain fewer, and milder, anthraquinone-containing plants—just cascara sagrada bark and rhubarb root, alongside barberry bark, raspberry leaf, fennel seed, golden seal root, lobelia herb, and smaller amounts of cayenne and ginger. In cases of mild constipation these will be very useful, but in the bowel cleanse programme they will be necessary in many cases since the IF2 formula—the drawing powder—may in certain circumstances cause bowel motions to slow down. Therefore, whether you feel that you need the extra help or not, I would never supply the IF2 drawing powder without a motility capsule of one of these specifications.

Drawing powder

There are various versions of the drawing formula. If you read Jensen's book, *Tissue Cleansing through Bowel Management*,[1] you will find a different recipe, but the idea is the same. In fact, nineteenth-century pioneer of the Natural Hygiene movement, Arnold Ehret, much admired by Dr Christopher, had his version as well, called the "intestinal broom"—which gives us a very good idea of what it was designed to do.

The one I use contains the following ingredients:

Powders of
– Marshmallow root
– Psyllium husks
– Fennel seeds
– Flax seeds (linseed)
– Bentonite clay
– Fruit pectin (apple or citrus)
– Activated charcoal (usually either sycamore or willow)

The formula combines the mucilaginous and demulcent properties, and the fibre, of marshmallow root, linseed and psyllium, together with the absorption capacity of bentonite clay, fruit pectin and activated charcoal, aided and assisted by the gas-dispersing and gut-relaxing properties of fennel seed.

A word of warning about flaxseed or linseed: if you buy a product with these in, make sure it has been vacuum-packed to guard against oxidation of the natural oils contained within the seeds. We do not want to introduce rancid oils into a detoxification programme. I make the formula up myself without the linseeds, and then supply these separately for those who want to grind them immediately prior to mixing.

Start with two servings in the first 3 or 4 days, rising to three for the next week, and reducing to two for the latter 3 or 4 days in a two-week programme. For this I find 100g of the powder sufficient, along with a supply of the motility capsules to ensure reliable transit.

So, the two-week bowel cleanse protocol that I routinely prescribe is as follows:

- If taking the IF1 route, first establish at least one motion daily by taking one capsule with the evening meal until a reliable motion is produced the following morning. You can increase to two or even three capsules if you need them to achieve this aim. Once you have got there, you can start on the IF2 powders.
- If taking the IF3 route, again take one capsule with your evening meal, rising to three or four if necessary during the cleanse, and start using the IF2 powder immediately.
- IF2—take 1 heaped teaspoon of the powders blended into full tumbler of water, twice daily BETWEEN meals—for example, mid-morning and mid-afternoon—for 3 or 4 days.
- Then increase the dose for the next 6 or 7 days to three times daily, the additional dose being taken in the evening before retiring.
- For the final 3 or 4 days, reduce back down to two doses daily, and then on the last day just one dose.
- The motility capsules can be adjusted as needed during the programme—if you find yourself getting too loose, reduce the number of capsules, or doses; if you feel you are becoming constipated, increase the dose or frequency.

IMPORTANT NOTE: the IF2 powder should ideally be blended into approximately 300ml water. The powders ABSORB moisture, so you may need more than this to ensure that, once inside you, they do not cause drying—and hence constipation. Ideally you should maintain a daily consumption of at least 2 litres of clean water during a detox programme. The most common mistake of people on a detox is to fail to hydrate adequately.

Bowel cleanse diet

It is not necessary to fast during the bowel cleanse, in fact it can be helpful to continue to eat, as that way the continuity of bowel motions is easier to maintain. If you are fasting, or want to fast, this is possible, but the use of the motility capsules will be all the more important as without the bulk of food, the peristalsis will slow down or even stop. See the end of this chapter for further specific advice on food intake during detoxification.

However, a clean, natural diet, predominantly plant-based, is strongly advised. Please refer to Chapter 4 for more guidance.

Colonics and enemas

These can be added into the programme and may serve to overcome the possible issue of constipation. If fasting, they are highly recommended. Since we are concerned here only with what we can accomplish in our own homes with simple equipment, I will leave colonic hydrotherapy out of the discussion and focus on self-administered enemas.

You will need to obtain an enema kit—basically a plastic bucket or bag with a hose leading from the bottom end, a tap near the distal end of the hose to turn the flow on and off, and a couple of cannulas to fit into the relevant orifices—most kits these days double as either rectal enema or vaginal douche. The vaginal canula is larger and equipped with irrigation holes all along its length and around its girth. The rectal cannula is smaller and equipped with just one hole at its tip.

The enema bag usually has a capacity of 2 litres, and can be filled with various solutions, the simplest of which is just plain water, but you can also make up herbal and nutritive teas and juices, depending on the action and affect required. Yellow dock root is a popular choice, as it has a mild stimulating action that contributes to the cleanse. You can add in dandelion root (also a mild aperient), barberry bark (a potent gastrointestinal antiseptic), or (if you can obtain and/or afford it) goldenseal, one of the best mucous membrane tonics and antiseptics in the herbal world. You can also use chlorella for cleansing, nourishing and assisting in the removal of heavy metal residues, or a soothing demulcent mix of mucilaginous herbs such as marshmallow root and slippery elm bark.

Prepare approximately 500ml (1 pint) of your chosen herb or herb mix by making a decoction, using 750ml water and 30g (1 oz) of the herb or herb mix. (This instruction is not relevant for chlorella, by the way, where you can simply add the powder or the juice to the total enema liquid.) Place the herbs and the water (the cleanest you can get—pure spring water, filtered or distilled) in a suitably sized pan and bring to the boil, the turn down to simmer with the lid on for 10 minutes. Once decocted, you should find you are able to strain out a good 500ml of the "tea". Let cool and then dilute to 1/4 total volume by adding 1.5 litres (3 pints) of suitably pure water. This gives 2 litres of fluid, which is the capacity of most enema bags, and you can now fill your bag for immediate use (do not pre-prepare and store for later use, e.g. in the fridge—the enema solution is best administered at room temperature or somewhere near, and as freshly made as possible).

The administration is best done as a "high enema" in my opinion. This is a technique of getting the enema solution right back around the colon as far as the ilio-caecal junction, the proximal end of the colon, and it does require some agility! Here is how to perform a high enema:

1. Ensure you have passed a bowel motion if you need to.
2. Hang your filled enema bag or bucket on something about the height of a shower hook or shower curtain rail—the gravity thus produced helps the flow. It is best to do this in the bath, as any spillage can then be washed down the drain.
3. Lying on your left side in the bath, insert the cannula carefully into the rectum. Cannulas specifically made for this application will be perfectly safe—but make sure you have attached the correct cannula—anything longer (the vaginal cannula is quite a bit bigger) risks rupturing the delicate tissues at the sigmoid/rectal flexure: the rectal cannula is made just short of the average rectal length. Exercise caution in any case and stop if you experience pain or discomfort.

That said, there is really very little danger of harm if you are using a proper kit—or they would not be allowed to sell it to you!
4. Open the tap to allow maybe a third of the liquid to enter your bowel. Because you are on your left side the enema solution will enter the sigmoid colon and then flow into the descending colon up to the splenic flexure (just underneath the ribcage on the upper left side of your abdomen).
5. Turn off the tap, and then shift onto your back, bringing your knees up, feet flat on the bath floor. Here's where being a bit flexible comes in: lift your pelvis off the floor of the bath so that you are in the yoga "bridge" pose, and now turn on the tap once more. Gravity should now act to push the liquid into the transverse colon—the bit that runs in a horizontal loop under your ribcage, to the hepatic flexure, in the upper-right abdomen.
6. Remain in the bridge pose for as long as is comfortable, and then shift round onto your right side. Turn on the tap to allow the remaining third of the solution to enter the colon. The fluid will now be pushed into your ascending colon, all the way up to the caecum.
7. Now hold the enema in place for as long as you can (practise to extend the time up to 10 or even 15 minutes), before removing the cannula, exiting the bath and releasing into the toilet pan. At this point it is probably prudent to state that the likelihood of not being able to hold the liquid for very long at the first few tries is quite high: hence the advice to use the bath to perform this routine. If this happens do not worry, simply use your shower to hose down the bath, and then yourself.

The coffee enema

Dr Jensen once joked that there is nothing wrong with coffee in a healing programme: it's just that people put it into the wrong hole! People do misunderstand the role of the coffee enema, however, and it is not my intention here to give full instruction in this advanced technique.

If you want to try a coffee enema please get appropriate practical input from a qualified naturopath. I once had to rescue a group of lay people who had attended a weekend naturopathic workshop and been instructed on the Saturday to each go home and perform a coffee enema. Three of the six participants did not return for the Sunday session; two of the remaining three contacted me the following week in a state of anxiety and some discomfort asking for appointments to help them overcome the "side-effects".

A coffee enema is not a "high" enema, like the one described in the previous section. You do not have to do any of the yoga poses or hold onto a huge amount of liquid for any length of time. The purpose of the coffee enema is actually to stimulate the liver. The coffee is absorbed through the colon lining into the mesenteric vein, where it is transported directly up to the liver, stimulating that organ to detoxify strongly, resulting in the rapid "dumping" of bile into the digestive tract, which can also be strongly stimulated through this method.

Bile, as we have seen, is not only a digestive fluid, but also an effluent, by which the products of liver detoxification are carried out of the system through the intestinal tract, and a significant laxative in its own right. It can be an exhilarating experience, but if you are not used to it, as our naturopathic participants found, it can be a little scary.

The coffee used is not regular stuff, by the way. Enema coffee must be fully organic in origin and be carefully roasted and prepared in order to retain the specialised phytochemistry that is required to do the trick. You can buy appropriately prepared coffee beans easily enough online these days. I don't want anyone putting this book down and going off to make a cup of instant coffee to introduce into their rectum!

The kidney flush

The kidney flush is nominally the simplest detox routine out of all of them, and in fact many people are already routinely performing a version of this without necessarily knowing it. In fact, any time you are feeling the need for a detox, but perhaps haven't got the time or the inclination to go for one of the more involved routines, such as bowel or liver, a few days of the kidney flush can serve to put you on top quite quickly.

Preparation

You will need:

- 1 lemon, juiced
- Tincture or powder of cayenne pepper
- Clean water (see Chapter 4)

- (Optional) Maple syrup
- (Optional) herbal "Kidney-Bladder" tea

The routine is performed first thing in the morning for 14 days. The various components are not accidental or random. In fact, they were first stipulated in naturopath Stanley Burroughs' "Master Cleanser" routine. This is a more far-reaching programme, consisting of a total fast throughout 21 days, using only this drink. In these terms the maple syrup serves to keep the metabolism boosted in the absence of solid foods. This, however, is an advanced routine, so for our purposes here we do not often recommend the syrup. For most people, one initial morning drink, backed up with the herbal kidney-bladder tea (see below), will suffice to form a perfectly manageable cleanse over a two-week period.

Lemons are the detox fruit *par excellence*. Interestingly, they also perform useful functions in the liver, in particular assisting with the task of rendering fat-soluble toxins water-soluble and helping to promote carbonate-rich secretions (to offset the acidity), which helps to maintain the correct environment in the duodenum—the area of the gastrointestinal tract into which the liver/gall bladder discharges bile.

Some naturopaths are not great fans of lemons, believing them to be acidifying, owing to their content of citric acid. Should they dig a little deeper however, they will find that upon processing in the body, the acid content actually resolves in favour of alkalinity. Lemons, in fact, are the arch-alkalisers among familiar and easy-to-access fruits. Limes, by the way, can also be used in this programme, and my personal favourite is to combine both.

I once treated a case of rheumatoid arthritis in a 40-year-old woman. When she arrived for her initial consultation, she announced that she had already made an appointment with a very well-known naturopath (now deceased), but that as there was a nine-month waiting list, she would see what could be accomplished in the short term by seeing me.

In additional to supplying her with an individualised herbal formula, I got her going on the basic detoxes and cleanses, including the kidney cleanse, which in addition to the lemon juice contained another supposedly controversial food—cayenne pepper, a member of the notorious Nightshade family, often contraindicated with arthritis.

The patient made excellent progress. Nonetheless, upon eventually attending her appointment with the naturopath, he was horrified to hear what I had been recommending. He said, "Take his herbs, but not his advice!" She became quite angry with me, asking me what I thought I was doing advising her to take these substances when she had a serious autoimmune arthritic condition. I gently asked her how she had fared on my detox programmes, whereupon she stopped suddenly in her tracks and thought, and then admitted that she had felt better than she had for a long time, and that the pain and inflammation had in fact substantially reduced. In fact, so great had been the improvement that she had almost reconsidered the need to see the famous and expensive naturopath at all.

To prepare the Kidney Flush, proceed as follows. First thing in the morning, prepare the following drink:

- Juice 1 lemon, and if you are feeling adventurous, 1 lime
- Add this to around a half litre of clean water
- Add either 10 drops of tincture of cayenne pepper, or a pinch of the raw powder
- You can add a dessertspoonful of maple syrup if you find the lemon too sour, but actually it's best to down the mix as it is and wrinkle up your nose instead!

Take your time drinking it down, though, for fear of causing discomfort to the stomach. A half hour after drinking this you can eat normally—although as with the bowel cleanse it is desirable to ensure a clean, natural diet for the duration of this cleanse.

Some might be concerned about the acidity of lemons on their teeth. My initial advice if this is the case is to drink the juice through a straw, but if even that seems undesirable, you can try substituting the lemon juice with apple cider vinegar.

You can also substitute ginger for the cayenne, if you feel cayenne is too hot for you. The role of cayenne in the mix is to act as a safe stimulant for the circulation, the kidneys and the adrenals—often also to break the habit of having that initial cup of coffee in the morning before any other food or drink. Many people find that it is quite sufficient to wake them up and get them going in the morning. However, in practice I will not use cayenne if:

- There is any sign of stomach discomfort or reflux
- The patient is suffering from facial acne or malar flushes on the face

- The patient is suffering from "toxic" headaches or signs of heat referred upward to the head region. Cayenne is a strong cerebral circulatory stimulant, but it may be too strong for some people.

The flush can also be taken as a warm or hot drink if desired, and a good variation is to add the lemon juice to an infused cup of fresh ginger tea—the ginger will substitute nicely for the cayenne for those who find the strong pungency difficult to take.

An optional—but highly recommended—addition to the cleanse is the kidney-bladder tea. Among herbs to choose for this are nettle leaf, dandelion leaf, celery seed, parsley root, horsetail herb, uva ursi leaf, cornsilk, goldenrod and wild carrot. One of my favourite blends is:

- Dandelion leaf — 2 parts
- Nettle leaf — 2 parts
- Uva ursi leaf — 1 part
- Horsetail herb — 1 part
- Goldenrod herb — 1 part
- Cornsilk or marshmallow leaf — 1 part
- Celery seed — ½ part

Infuse for 10–15 minutes, drink 2 or 3 cups daily.

Lastly, in relation to the vulnerability of the kidneys in respect of their supposed inability to regenerate, I want to mention some measures that have been seen to reverse even dangerously severe loss of kidney function (known as chronic kidney disease, or CKD).

The first of these is the herb nettle, but it is not to the usual part of the plant—the leaf—to which we look, nor even the root—much in favour for the treatment of the prostate gland; but the *seed*. Nettle is a largely unsung Western "adaptogen", meaning that it bolsters stamina and vitality in the face of stress. Much of the detriment accruing to chronic stress involves the draining and weakening of the kidneys, which are, as already mentioned, the seat of our vitality, seen from a traditional medicine point of view. Nettle seed has been associated with several anecdotal reversals of CKD and is an excellent choice where kidney function is challenged by stress and exhaustion.

Second, the medicinal mushroom *Cordyceps militaris* has a very similar profile in helping to apparently rebuild the kidneys once depleted and reduced by chronic stress and inflammation.

And lastly, barley grain: some readers may be old enough to remember the use of barley water as a tonic for strengthening in convalescence. Barley grain, either soaked in water and taken as a drink with lemon juice, or cooked in stews and casseroles, is a traditional remedy for flagging kidneys and overworked adrenals.

The liver flush

There are a few naturopathic routines for clearing out the liver and gall bladder. Some are specialised responses to actual liver/gall bladder complaints such as biliary colic and cholecystitis (inflammation of the gall bladder). One very famous protocol is the Andreas Moritz "amazing liver and gall bladder cleanse", involving the use of Epsom salts. Although I have deep respect for Moritz's work, I am not inclined to recommend this routine to all and sundry, having a few times been involved in rescuing people who should not really have been advised to undertake it. I think that as part of a professionally directed programme, with all safety parameters assessed and monitored, this routine can be powerfully healing, however here I am more concerned to give people simple and safe tools that can be used in cure, but perhaps most effectively in prevention, and so we will not concern ourselves with these more powerful methods.

The routine that I know and love and have been performing at the time of writing regularly three or four times a year for the last nearly 50 years, is also known as the "Polarity Liver Flush", as it was promoted by Dr Randolph Stone, the architect of Polarity Therapy, which I mentioned briefly in my preface. Stone also advocated a specific herbal tea as part of this cleanse, known affectionately by his students as *Polaritea*, which is very similar to the "detox tea" outlined below.

I was familiar with the liver flush protocol from my very first engagement with Natural Healing in my very early 20s, so I was delighted to find it again when I studied Polarity Therapy, and again upon studying herbal medicine with Dr Schulze. Here is the routine in all its glory.

Preparation

For this 10-day routine you will need to prepare daily each morning:

- 1 whole lemon, juiced—you can actually use the entire lemon here, not just the internal juice, but pulp, pith, rind, seeds and all
- Thumb-sized portion of fresh ginger root
- 1 large clove of garlic
- 1 tablespoon of organic, cold-pressed olive oil
- 300ml freshly juiced organic apples (best to juice for the occasion, but I have often found shop-bought organic fresh-pressed juice serves perfectly well)
- Pinch of cayenne pepper powder (optional)

Start first thing by drinking a large tumbler of fresh, clean water. This is to ensure that there is enough fluid with which to manufacture the bile that is going be needed to flush the liver effectively.

Then blend the above ingredients in a jug blender. Drink the mix down (it actually tastes quite good), and then begin preparing a herbal "Detox Tea" using all or any of the following ingredients:

- Dandelion root (strongly recommended)
- Burdock root
- Yellow dock root
- Dandelion greens
- Nettle leaf
- Cleavers herb
- Red clover blossoms

These are all blood-cleansing "alterative" herbs. Dandelion is the most useful general-purpose liver dredger, and the other herbs variously cover liver, kidneys and lymph.

In addition, you can add some warming spices, such as ginger root, cinnamon bark, fennel seed, fenugreek seed and liquorice root—use these in much smaller quantities as they can be strongly pungent. These help to maintain blood sugar and energy in what is actually going to be an extension of your overnight fast for the first two hours of your waking day.

Here is an illustration of a well-rounded and suitably powerful "detox" tea blend that we prepare in our own dispensary:

The Natural Centre

17 Herb Detox Tea – 100g

Ingredients: *Arctium lappa*(Burdock root), *Arctostaphylos uva ursi* (Bearberry leaf), *Cinnamomum zeylannicum* (Cinnamon bark), *Citrus aurantium* (Orange peel), *Elettaria Cardamomum* (Cardamom pods), *Foeniculum vulgare* Fennel seed), *Galium aparine* (Cleavers herb), *Glycyrrhiza glabra* (Liquorice root), *Juniperus communis* (Juniper berries), *Rumex crispus* (Dock root), *Szygium aromaticum* (Cloves), *Tabebuia impetiginosa* (Pau d'Arco), *Taraxacum officinalis rad.* (Dandelion root), *Trifolium pratense* (Red Clover flowers), *Trigonella foenum-graecum* (Fenugreek seed), *Urtica dioica* (Nettle leaf), *Zingiber officinalis* (Ginger)

Figure 4. The 17-Herb detox tea.

Prepare these herbs in a large saucepan, using 30g of the combined herbs to 750ml (1.5 pints) of clean water (preferably distilled). Bring to a boil and then turn down the heat and simmer with the lid on for 10 minutes.

Strain out the herbs and pour the liquid into a large mug, which you can now start to drink—the hotter the better. Meanwhile replace the used herbs in the pan, add another 500ml water, and repeat the process. Drink AT LEAST 2 full mugs of this tea over the following 2-hour period. It will help to be at home for this, as some of these herbs are strong diuretics and you will almost certainly want to visit the loo a couple of times!

For this reason, it may be advisable to choose a period of 10 days when you can be mainly at home. You can work from home and carry out most of your daily activities perfectly well during this cleanse, and once the initial 2 hours is done, you should be able to go out and carry on as normal. If your place of work is reasonably near your home, you can if you wish prepare the herbal decoction and put it in a thermos flask to take with you—however if you use public transport be wary of being caught short on longer journeys! The other caution is not to leave it too long between drinking the initial smoothie and taking the detox tea—20 minutes is optimal, at a stretch 30, but longer than that and you will start to lose the advantage. After 20 minutes the liver will be discharging—"dumping"—bile at an accelerated rate, and the tea will be needed to help flush that through the digestive tract.

Tips and cautions

- Diet, again, should be clean, natural and predominantly plant-based. See the end of this chapter for further specific advice on food intake during detoxification. Breaking the initial "fast" after the 2 hours of the flush should be done gently: fruit is ideal for this, and then if still hungry something more substantial may be taken 30 minutes after the fruit.
- While performing this flush it is necessary to maintain optimum hydration of around 2 litres daily of water. This is because the flush does drain fluids at an accelerated rate, both via liver and kidneys.
- The flush usually proceeds smoothly with no adverse reactions or aggravations, although there can be just one day when you may feel somewhat sluggish: headaches, tiredness and even slight nausea may be experienced temporarily on day 4 of the routine. This is so often the case that it might be worth scheduling a "duvet day" for it in advance! The advice is to rest, drink plenty of fresh, clean water and herbal teas, keep warm and eat lightly if at all. Whatever you do, DO NOT take paracetamol or any other pharmaceutical pain relief. The symptoms are caused by be the temporary increase of circulating toxins in the blood stream and will pass quickly if you take the suggested advice.
- Sometimes people say, "I feel so good on this I'd like to keep doing it! Can I continue for another week or so?" Don't. That's all. You can repeat the cleanse every 3 to 4 months—in fact it is strongly advised that you do, but it is not necessary to prolong the cleanse. Ensure you have planned your "re-entry" to normal life and resolve to repeat the experience 3 or 4 times a year as routine maintenance. Once you have done one 10-day stretch, the repeats can even be shorter—5 days is a good interim period. But ensure one 10-day cleanse per year.
- You can even do a one-off day cleanse if you have a day when you feel that you might benefit from it: I have one patient who, since using the cleanse to help him through a cancer treatment, now routinely does a liver flush every Friday—and swears by it.

The lymphatic system

It is my usual custom to recommend lymph moving and clearing measures throughout the detox period. Many of these measures are standard health-enhancing practices that can also be added into your daily routine even when not detoxing, and include:

Dry skin brushing

(See also the section below on skin for detailed instructions.) This practice, done daily, serves to continuously remove dead skin and unblock pores, as well as to stimulate the peripheral blood and lymph circulation.

Hydrotherapy

This can consist either of simple contrast showers done in your own bathroom, or saunas followed by cold plunges, steam rooms, sitz baths and so on. These will be discussed in the skin section below but are also powerful ways of moving and detoxifying lymph.

Exercise

It is well-known that rebounding on a mini trampoline is the optimum exercise for the lymph system, but any form of exercise is beneficial. Other strong contenders are hatha yoga and swimming.

Deep breathing

The thoracic duct, the central lymph reservoir, is located just in front of the thoracic spine and runs through the diaphragm. When you breathe in deeply it has the effect of massaging this channel and thus acts like a pump to assist in the circulation of lymph.

Bodywork

There are some specific styles of bodywork that address the lymph. One of the best known is manual lymphatic drainage (MLD), but within Polarity Therapy, for example, there are other lymph-moving and -draining practices. For these, obviously, you will need to find and book a professional practitioner.

Diet

Food choices should steer away from "the usual suspects"—sugar, especially, and "white carbs" (white flour products, biscuits, cakes, pastries), milk products, highly heated fats and processed foods, and alcohol. See the cleanse-diet suggestions at the end of this chapter.

Herbs

Herbs can also be used to assist in lymph cleansing. Probably the best-known herb in this respect is cleavers—otherwise called bedstraw or sticky willy. It grows prolifically in Northern Europe in the springtime and is very much associated with "spring cleaning" for the body. One of the best ways to prepare it, should you be doing your detox in the spring, is by cold infusion: grab a handful of the herb, rub it between your hands briefly and drop it into a tumbler or large mug. Top up with clean water and let stand overnight. In the morning strain out the liquid and drink.

However, probably the best-known herb for the purposes of lymph cleansing is a plant that few (unless they have studied it) associate specifically with the lymph at all—echinacea. In its traditional context echinacea is regarded as a "lymphatic alterative", which means that it cleanses the lymph. We usually see it as an "immune booster" for use in the treatment of colds and 'flu. Perhaps, if our understanding of herbs is a little more sophisticated, we might characterise it as an "immunomodulator".

But think for a moment: if lymph is responsible for circulating immune cells, then echinacea's action on immunity is probably going to impact the health of the lymph. In fact, one of echinacea's most celebrated actions is to increase the production of phagocytes—or macrophages. As we have already mentioned, these "big eaters" have the job of gobbling up debris and removing it from circulation. If that does not suggest lymph-cleansing, I don't know what does.

There are a few myths surrounding the correct way of using echinacea, however, with some suggesting that is not safe for ongoing continuous use. Australian herbalist Kerry Bone has pretty much disproved this idea and is a great advocate (and personal advertisement) for the regular daily use of this herb. The only contraindication to extended use is pregnancy—and even here it can be used in short bursts if needed.

The skin

I have already laid the foundations for understanding the importance of the skin in detoxification. The skin is a permeable membrane—it secretes, via perspiration, and of course it also absorbs, selectively. It is also our physical outer sheath and boundary, and it needs to be maintained in correct health and balance. It carries the peripheral circulatory channels, both blood and lymph, and, by opening and closing the vascular channels, as well as the pores, it regulates temperature.

Here are the details on how to take care of it. These practices can be adopted as lifestyle measures, or they can be prioritised when undergoing a dedicated detoxification programme.

Dry skin brushing

Skin brushes may be readily purchased these days on the internet. Use one with natural bristles—usually coconut—and if possible, get one with a long handle, so you reach the difficult-to-reach parts like the mid-back.

Starting at the extremities, brush in small circles, working up toward the torso. Do the arms and legs first. Then work around the buttocks into the small of the back, and upwards to the flanks and ribcage. At this point it will usually be necessary to change to working from above; get the shoulders done, then move down to the scapulae and between. When this is done work around to the front of the torso, with gentle movements around the breasts and chest, and finishing up with large circular sweeps around the abdomen and umbilicus, in the direction of peristaltic flow—that's the direct the bowels move in—clockwise.

You can do your face, but I advise a smaller and softer brush for this—you can get special facial brushes.

DO NOT brush over any skin rashes—eczema, psoriasis or acne—or over cuts or grazes. Let these heal before attempting to brush.

This routine may be performed every morning before bathing or showering. It needs to be done when dry. When you first start doing it watch carefully as you brush—you will often see clouds of dead skin flying off! This effect will slow down as you keep doing it, as you will have successfully exfoliated to a high degree. Dry skin brushing exfoliates, especially removing debris from the all-important pores, and stimulates peripheral blood and lymph circulation.

One of my abiding memories of listening to Dr Jensen lecture way back in 1978 was the moment, when extolling the virtues of dry skin brushing, he rolled up his trouser leg to expose his calf, in order to demonstrate that regular skin brushing can give you "the skin of a baby"—even at his ripe age of around 70 at the time. I was actually sitting in the front row, literally right at his feet as he was on a 3-foot-high platform, so I had the best view. I can verify the truth of his assertion.

Hydrotherapy

There are a number of ways in which you can engage with the very powerful practice of using alternating hot and cold water as part of a regular health maintenance programme, or indeed simply as an adjuvant treatment in a detox. You may have to get creative about this if, for example, you do not have a particularly powerful shower in your home.

You can also outsource this aspect of your healing by using a hydrotherapy spa if you happen to have one in your neighbourhood. If you are lucky enough to have a sauna in your home then you have a wonderful resource that I also encourage you to share with others! Turkish baths, steam baths, hot rooms, cold plunges, sitz baths and post-treatment massages are all bonuses to visiting a good spa, so take full advantage if you are able to.

But what I specifically want to cover here is the usual home option of contrast showers, which can be taken every day if desired, and do not generally involve additional expense or travel.

It is important that you get your standard ablutions done before going to the hot–cold routine, so wash yourself and shampoo your hair (preferably using clean natural products of course). Then turn down the hot water. You can go gently with this—even a lukewarm shower will contrast sufficiently if you are not used to the cold—but try to push the envelope, each time gong a little colder. I suggest at first around 20 seconds cold, then go back to warm or hot for one minute. Then go back to lukewarm, cool or cold, as suggested taking it a little further, for another 20 or 30 seconds. You can perform the alternation up to six times in the course of one shower.

I like to recommend ending on cold, as I personally find that the most bracing, but if you are suffering with fatigue and depletion, or any rheumatic condition, standard advice is to end on warm (not hot). Upon leaving the shower wrap up and keep warm.

I am personally doing this a little differently these days, so if you have the courage, try this. After showering normally, washing and shampooing, turn the hot tap off quickly and dowse yourself in a sudden blast of cold. Stand under the cold shower for a full minute, rising to two minutes once you get used to it. The cold will force you to breath very deeply, and when you get out you will feel super-invigorated. These days my day does not start until I have done this: once done, I am ready for anything.

Hot water immersion stimulates circulation, but tends to relax and slow down respiration, whereas cold water does the opposite—it stimulates respiration and slows down circulation. Except that, more accurately, what it does is drive the circulation deeper into the body, away from the periphery. Alternating hot and cold does a kind of pumping action—driving the blood deeper, then pulling it back to the surface, and back and forth for as long as you keep doing it. This is very invigorating and cleansing to both blood and lymph, and it also means that the blood enters the deeper structures of the body, particularly the major joints, delivering oxygen and nutrients, and draining and removing wastes, over and over again.

Ice-cold immersions, of the kind advocated by Dutch health guru Wim Hof (the Ice Man), work specifically according to this principle. The revitalising blood is driven deep into the body, maximising its healing and nourishing principles, and the practice also serves to approximate the effect of therapeutic hypothermia, which has been shown to be a very powerful healing tool in injury and some chronic disease patterns including myocardial infarction (heart attack). If you are really hard-core, then go and buy a personal cold immersion tub—and don't forget to add ice to every immersion!

Lastly, something you can do to speed up the healing of traumatic injury, specifically of the musculoskeletal system, is to apply the alternating hot and cold treatments locally, directing the shower head at the affected part and again switching between hot and cold for several cycles. In addition to speeding up the healing, it also works as a highly effective method of pain relief. I find it particularly useful to recommend on arthritic joints.

If treating the musculoskeletal system, particularly, it can also help to have a "deep heat" herbal tissue-repair oil or embrocation at hand, to apply immediately upon exiting the shower.

Topical treatments: Clay, salt and oils

There is much written about the healing properties of mud and clay, and it is not my intention to go deeply into this subject. The "what, where, when and how" of these treatments need careful evaluation, and it is best to seek individual advice. In my opinion there are few more relaxing and healthful ways of applying these treatments than getting a suitably qualified therapist to do it for you.

Clothes and topical products

In terms of skin care, it matters what kinds of topical products you use, as of course also what kinds of fabrics you wear, and what you wash them in. In fact, when buying household cleaning products of any kind remember that these are one of the most easily overlooked sources of toxicity in our modern lives. Try to find ecologically sound and sustainable versions of products such as laundry liquids, dishwasher tablets and other necessities—they are out there, but you will need to focus your search to find them. At all costs "natural" is the watchword, but remember the discussion in Chapter 1 about that word: do not take anything for granted—research the product and ask the relevant questions.

In terms of fabric, cotton, linen and wool are basically safe, but ensure these are not blended with synthetics such as nylon, rayon, lycra and polyester. Bamboo if sustainably grown and properly processed is fine; hemp and nettle are fast gaining ground as ecologically sound and kind to the skin. Remember, the skin needs to breathe and perspire.

Do NOT use: chemical deodorants or antiperspirants, standard chemical toiletries or cosmetics, and especially DO NOT USE chemical sunscreen: this has been demonstrated to be carcinogenic, and in some cases the sun has been blamed for skin cancers in situations where it may very well have been the sunscreen or tanning product that caused the problem. If you think about it, to baste yourself in a chemical cocktail and then lay yourself out like a side of lamb to roast sounds like a recipe for skin cancer—to me at least. Herbal alternatives are jojoba oil (SPF 16), carrot seed oil (SPF 35–40) and raspberry seed oil (SPF 25–50).

Lastly, remember that your skin is kept healthy not just by what you choose to put on it, but also what you choose to put into yourself. Food intake and medicines will also make a difference, and in terms of the latter there are several herbs that have a clear affinity to the skin—examples include burdock root, mountain grape root, red clover flowers, marigold flowers, and cleavers. The skin is often the outward-facing barometer of internal conditions.

The lungs

We will be looking closely at what we can do to protect and heal the lungs in the chapter on Ambient Air, below. As I have already suggested, it is a highly topical subject, and we need to be paying it special attention at this time.

For the present discussion, let us just emphasise deep breathing practices, but also caution against domestic chemical sprays, deodorants, air-fresheners, perfumes and cleaning agents—and above all, CIGARETTE SMOKE: commercial tobacco manufacturing produces a cocktail of some of the most hazardous chemical toxins available. Amongst the Indian tribes of North, Central and South America, tobacco is revered as a healing Master Plant. Europeanised commercial interests have turned it into an addictive, health-destroying monster.

Additional detox advice

Food intake

I have already given basic advice about this, but it does bear repeating as it is one of the most common questions that I get asked when prescribing detox solutions. The overall thrust and character of the protocols in this chapter are towards simple regimes that are safe and easy to perform at home, with or without specialist help. In general terms then, it is not necessary to fast, nor to go on an unduly restricted diet. The basic rules may be summarised as follows:

- Largely vegan/plant-based (no meat or dairy), but avoid "plant-based" processed foods, which can be just as bad if not worse (see next chapter).
- Avoid if possible: sugar, refined carbohydrates, alcohol, coffee, black tea (green and white are OK), vinegar (except cider vinegar), yeast (including yeasted bread).
- Plenty of: fresh produce, raw or lightly steamed vegetables, greens, fruit (but separate fruit from vegetables, don't eat together at the

same meal), whole grains (rice, millet, buckwheat, quinoa), nuts and seeds, sprouted legumes and seeds (can sprout your own or get ready-sprouted from some wholefood outlets).
- Fluids: 2 litres filtered or distilled water daily; 1 superfood smoothie (see below) daily; herbal teas and grain coffees. Juices (see below), but do not buy these ready-juiced unless you can guarantee the processing used has not resulted in oxidation of the product.
- Supplements (optional): Ω 3, 6, 9 oils (e.g. flax, hempseed). Vitamin C—1000mg per day in supplement or food format. "Superfood" powder, e.g. The Natural Centre "Rainbow Blend", or Dr Schulze's Superfood—organic, plant-based vitamin and mineral supplement, blended with water and fresh fruits.
- The Blended Salad (green smoothie): based on Robert O. Young's pH Miracle recipe, is a favourite for detox diets. Simply place a good handful of green leaves (spinach, spring greens, rocket, watercress etc.) with a short section of cucumber, a celery stalk, half a bell pepper and half an avocado, into a jug blender and cover with the cleanest water you can access (see Chapter 4). Add lemon or lime juice to taste, as well as half a clove of fresh garlic and a small piece of fresh grated ginger. A pinch of a good-quality mineral-rich salt (e.g. Celtic or Himalayan) can set it off nicely, and if you really want to fortify it, add some supergreens, such as the Dr Schulze Superfood blend (see above). Blend and drink.

Food is the subject of the next chapter and will introduce the basic rules of how to choose and prioritise foods in your diet. If you can train yourself to eat a natural diet, as free as possible from the ubiquitous threats of commercialised food production, then you will not have so much work to do when it comes to your detox initiatives. Juicing will also be discussed and can be a radical assistant to successful detoxing.

When to detoxify

The routines in the chapter can be repeated regularly a few times a year if desired. It's a good idea to schedule detox opportunities for yourself at key points during the year. These should, as already discussed, preferably coincide with periods of more home-based activity, but once you are proficient you may find that you can easily detox in the midst of your ordinary working routine.

Good times to set up routine detoxes are change of seasons—particularly the transition from winter to spring, and again from summer to autumn. Another good time is after a traditional "celebration", which may have involved inadvisable party foods and beverages. Christmas and New Year are the most obvious examples, but there may be others in your life.

Also useful is any time you are starting to feel "under the weather", "coming down" with something, or just overwhelmed and "toxic". Even a short period of detoxing using maybe the kidney or liver flush can sometimes get you back on top quite quickly.

As an aside here, I personally believe that "coming down with a cold" is very simply your body's way of activating a spontaneous detox, and is often a signal that things have gotten "backed up", and the detox and elimination channels are overwhelmed. The phlegm that is produced in copious amounts during such events is full of the debris of immune cells (phagocytes) that have been used to "fight the infection" (i.e. to clear out the accumulation).

Lastly, and this may sound counter-intuitive, learn to ENJOY detoxing! If you go into it thinking it's going to be a chore, all about deprivation and starvation, then you will find it much more difficult. Once you have had the experience of how much extra vitality these practices will give you, and how quickly your usual aches and pains start to reduce or disappear, then all you have to do is remind yourself how great you are going to feel as a result of your routine detox "holidays" and start to look forward to them.

The one-month detox programme

This programme covers all systems in an easy-to-do one-month programme and is something I use for many clients where detox is required to engage with chronic health issues. I never introduce it at the first meeting, preferring to work on the basics of diet, lifestyle, exercise and so forth for at least the first month of treatment, alongside a "preparatory", individualised herbal prescription aimed at general toning and harmonisation of the whole system.

Once I give the go-ahead, and the patient has agreed and found a suitable stretch of time in their routines that will allow them to complete the programme comfortably, we supply the relevant herbal products and walk them through the process.

Finding a suitable period does not mean that you must not be working or doing anything in your life: it simply means that your progress is not going to be impeded by other events and activities that may intervene to disrupt or otherwise make it difficult—such as Christmas (unless you prefer not to indulge in the usual excess of the season!), family celebrations and parties, travelling for work, and holidays: it is best not to detox on holiday unless you really feel that is how you want to spend your time away. Most, however, prefer to "enjoy" themselves in more conventional ways!

The programme looks like this:

Weeks 1 and 2:

- Kidney flush supported with a Kidney/Bladder tea.
- Bowel cleanse routine—enemas or colonics can also be added in this phase.
- Hydration, exercise, skin brushing and hydrotherapy as standard daily practices.

Weeks 3 and 4:

- Liver flush supported by the Detox tea.
- Lymph cleansing herbal tea or tincture.
- Hydration, exercise, skin brushing and hydrotherapy as standard daily practices.

Herbal products required:

- Cayenne tincture drops
- Bowel cleanse kit—motility capsules and drawing powder
- Kidney/bladder tea
- Detox tea
- Lymph cleanse tincture

5-Day "fast-track" detox

If you do not have time to spread this process out over a month, or even two weeks, you can try this 5-day routine:

Prepare the evening before by eating early, and lightly.

Day 1:

- On awakening, prepare and drink the Kidney Flush.
- Half an hour later have a light breakfast—fruit is ideal, or even some steamed green vegetables.
- Lunch can be a salad, or more steamed vegetables, plus if you like a small serving of an appropriate gluten-free grain—my favourites are quinoa or wholegrain Basmati rice.
- Drink plenty of fresh clean water all throughout the day—up to 3 litres—and herbal teas, preferably of a cleansing variety—nettle is ideal.
- Dinner again should be early (around 6pm) and similar to lunch.
- End the day with a relaxing herbal tea, such as chamomile, passionflower, skullcap or lemon balm.

Day 2:

- Day 2 is much as Day 1 up until lunch time, but lunch is going to be your last meal for 48 hours: from lunchtime Day 2 until lunch time Day 4 you will be on fluids only.
- Drink your daily quota of water plus any herbal teas that you fancy for the remainder of the day. You can also drink juices, provided that they are fresh-juiced—that means you juice them yourself!
- End the day with the sleepy-time relaxing tea.

Day 3:

- Begin Day 3 with the Liver Flush. For simplicity take either decocted dandelion root for the detox tea, or even simpler, a strong infusion of nettle tea. Have at least 2 large mugs of the tea in the two hours following the initial liver flush smoothie.
- You can in fact opt to drink the detox teas for the whole day, interspersed with plenty of water.
- Rest as much as possible: don't be tempted to do the washing, the house-cleaning, the shopping (why? You're fasting!) or running around after the kids. It's actually a great idea to negotiate with your nearest and dearest that you can take this time OFF. You can sell it to them by saying you are making sure that you have the strength and vitality to carry on caring for them for the next 12 months!

- Line up some great books, inspirational films or videos, meditate or pray, write in your journal, and so forth. You may feel bored and need things to do, so make them count: you are detoxing from the everyday chores of life too, so don't apologise for indulging some of your favourite activities, such as drawing or painting, writing poetry, playing music. I have a beautiful and very expensive guitar that I hardly ever give myself permission to play: this is an ideal opportunity. Whatever you do, DO NOT WORK. Day 3 is the pinnacle of the detox. Give yourself permission to take a complete holiday from everyday life and chores. You are, effectively, on retreat.

Day 4:

- Day 4 can begin with either Liver or Kidney Flush, as you choose.
- At lunchtime, prepare yourself a "blended salad" (see inset box).
- Dinner (6pm) can be a feast of steamed green vegetables or a tossed green salad. Add lightly roasted nuts and seeds if you feel you need some protein.

Day 5:

- Begin with the Kidney Flush.
- Lunch is the blended salad again.
- Dinner is the feast mentioned in Day 4, but hey, you can reintroduce grains here too!

The next day try and be true to the experience and don't rush to "retox". You can eat and drink normally—but cleanly. Try to use this experience as a reset—at least for a week or so. I once broke a fast on a diet of sandwiches, chocolate and beer: it is something I will never try again—an informative "experience", but not recommended!

You will have noticed that this routine contains a short fast in its midst. Because of the care that is taken in both entry to, and exit from the fast, it is quite safe for anyone to try, but care is needed if you are diabetic. In fact, fasting is good for diabetics, but it must be appropriately prepared for—get practised at shorter fasts before attempting longer or deeper ones—and conducted under close monitoring until you get used to it. More will be given on fasting in the next chapter.

Sample detox diary

When working with people on detoxification I frequently recommend that they keep a record of what happens on a day-to-day basis, by which they can assess the progress they are making. The following sample is for a fictional patient suffering with constipation, skin outbreaks (acne) and fatigue, on a 10-day liver detox:

Day	Bowel motions	Urination	Energy	Skin
1	0 – constipated	Dark yellow, 4 ×	3/10	Old outbreak persisting
2	1 – hard to pass	Still dark, but 5 ×	4/10	No change
3	1 – a little easier	Lighter, 5–6 ×	4/10	Start of some new lesions
4	2 – 1 slightly loose	Lighter, 5–6 ×	5/10	New heads developing
5	3 × very loose	Very frequent 7–8 ×	3/10	Accelerated outbreak
6	2 × more normal	Similar 6–7 ×	6/10	Spots starting to clear up
7	2 × after meals	5–6 × normal colour	6/10	Clear-up continues
8	× normal motion	6–7 ×	7/10	No new heads developing
9	2 × normal motion	6–7 ×	8/10	Clearing nicely
10	3 × normal motion	6–7 ×	8/10	Mostly clear, good skin tone

Figure 5. Sample detox diary.

You can choose to add more detail if you like—include a basic food diary, or at least how many times you ate on each day; other activities, e.g. exercise, sleep, work patterns, stressful episodes, other symptoms (whether transitory, or exacerbations of existing minor symptoms), and so forth.

The example in this table conforms to a pattern often seen, which is that for the first few days there is not a lot of improvement, and then a short period about half way through (day 4 or 5) when things seem to go worse, but then quite rapidly better, with energy levels potentially doubling over the rest of the detox period.

Keeping a record of your achievement does two things: it acts as encouragement—you are getting somewhere! It can also highlight other issues you may need to focus upon. For example, if you also record food intake, it may become very obvious that your reactions to certain foods are highly instructive, for better or for worse.

It also potentially provides a road map for future detox assignments, although here we need to sound a note of caution: the next time you run the protocol you might find it is dramatically different. This often happens if you don't notice much the first time, but the second occasion really puts you through the ringer! Or maybe you have a huge and highly significant improvement the first time, but the second time doesn't seem to produce much of an effect.

The variables in these situations are almost too complex to calculate, although they make good material for discussion at follow-up consultations, and may serve to bring other issues into awareness. One way or another, there is always something to learn from every individual detox.

Endnote

1. Jensen, B. (2011). *Tissue Cleansing through Bowel Management* (Escondido: Bernard Jensen Enterprises).

CHAPTER FOUR

Food and drink

We live in an age where there is no shortage of advice when it comes to food and eating. It spills out of every social media platform from a motley mixture of health gurus and celebrity doctors, supported by a never-ending range of must-have products, pills and potions, generating healthy profits for these individuals. However, if you were to pay close attention to all of it you would discover quite quickly that it can be highly contradictory and confusing.

Where one teaching extols the benefits of whole foods, for example, another advocates eating white rice because the "lectins" in the "brown" parts of the grain are indigestible and inflammation-promoting. Set against the sharp rise in people choosing veganism (or "plant-based"), encouraged by the ubiquity of vegan ethics and the environmental commentary (cows cause global warming), are the keto and paleo factions, which while not prohibitively carnivorous, are extremely difficult to commit to if you do not eat animal products.

Adding to the problem of "what to eat", however, is that the promoters of many of these systems and protocols rarely make themselves available for *personal* advice when things get confusing or difficult, often leaving something of a mess for practitioners such as myself to sort out.

There are a handful of systems that work on the basis of individual assessment. Dr Peter d'Adamo's *Eat Right 4 Your Type* is a system based on blood type as the indicator of what you should or should not be eating. The system has merit, as it is the closest that a conventional scientific understanding comes to a constitutional analysis of food preferences, but there are also some problems: the *choice* to be vegetarian when your O-type predicts you will not do so well on this can be conflicting to some people, while those who are told that their A-type blood means that eating animal-derived products is not good for them may feel similarly disadvantaged. It is important to remember that there are potentially many factors other than diet that come into play to cause "problems" in any constitution, for example the robustness of the individual digestive process itself (see later).

Then we have the weight loss systems. Again, they can be proliferous and confusing. One, however, caught my eye a long time ago and is worthy of mention. Based on the idea of "food combining", Harvey and Marilyn Diamond's classic, *Fit for Life*, served me well in the advice I was giving patients, mainly because it was not so much about the WHAT of eating, but the HOW and the WHEN. Mealtime Hygiene is a topic that we will be introducing in these pages as part of a manifesto for correct eating and has much in common with the basic notions of food combining. As weight-loss protocols these systems work by regulating and optimising metabolism, not by starving and depriving it.

Another system emanating from the weight-loss cohorts, but one which I rate highly, is that of my colleague Pippa Campbell in her book, *Eat Right, Lose Weight*.[1] Pippa discusses a range of metabolic types based on key processing organs and outlines the typical challenges of each, assessed by means of a simple questionnaire, and giving coherent and easy-to-follow advice on each type in terms of preferred food types and eating strategies. I for example fall into her "Adrenal" type, and on reading her advice it seemed immediately intuitive to me and reflected the way I have in fact over the years, through experience, preferred to manage my own diet.

Taking bio-individuality into account, it is sometimes a good idea to obtain personalised information about your digestive and metabolic profile, by visiting an appropriately-trained professional practitioner—nutritionist, naturopath, etc. As a practitioner I tend to rely on traditional medicine diagnoses and Iridology for this, and they have rarely failed me. If you are more "scientifically" inclined you might go for genomic and metabolic lab testing, which aims to give information based on genetic profiling. Functional Medicine labs can be accessed either by the lay individual, or through nutritionists and other practitioners who hold accounts with these facilities for the benefit of their patients. I myself do occasionally commission FM testing where I assess there is a need for that specific information.

It should go without saying that if you have chronic digestive difficulties, or in fact any other issue that fails to resolve spontaneously, you probably need to consult a knowledgeable professional—a herbalist, nutritionist or naturopath—and get an assessment. The advice given in these pages is of a general nature but can be deployed by anyone with a need to experiment in making improvements in their health. In many cases simple measures will have huge benefits, but refinements may also be possible with expert help.

What is food?

American journalist and Harvard professor Michael Pollan famously summarised a manifesto for eating in the soundbite, "Eat food, not too much, mainly plants". The first part of this phrase is maybe the most telling: much of what people are offered as food in supermarkets is not, in fact, food. It has little to do with the natural foods that our grandparents, and even our parents (if you are as old as I am) grew up on. It is *produced*—processed—often using high temperatures, which chemically alter the original starting material, flavoured, preserved and "enhanced", packaged to the hilt in materials that have frequently been found to "migrate" into the contents, and sold in bulk by means of brash advertising campaigns.

I was involved for eleven years in the wholefood industry in the UK. This movement had its origins in what I like to call the cultural revolution of the 1960s. Sometimes referred to as "Back to Nature", it was very much influenced by the influx of health modalities from the East, including traditional Chinese medicine, macrobiotics, and the Indic traditions of Yoga and Ayurveda, which were also highly influential in the Western cultural phenomenon known as the "hippie" movement. Essentially, it promoted the idea that food, wherever or however you found it, was best sourced as close to its natural state as possible. The more processing that took place, the less likely it was to be a wholesome product; but it also came with an *energetic* perspective on food—that is to say, it had an eye on the inherent vitality of food, and how it served individuals by reference to their own energetic deficiencies or surpluses.

One of the drawbacks of the movement, however, was that a lot of the food that was served (at least in the circles I moved in) was indigestible to most ordinary individuals—compact, dense, pudding-like slabs of stuff that challenged the strongest of digestive tracts—and mine was one of the strongest, according to my mother, who always declared I had a "cast iron" stomach.

However, the failure of twenty-something English idealists to translate their ecological fervour into culinary prowess should not invalidate the general idea, which is that we should be careful before we arrogate to ourselves the power to improve upon Nature, whatever or whomever you perceive that entity to be. I hold the same basic article of faith in relation to herbal medicines, preferring simple, traditional preparations and extractions over the encapsuled, compressed and refined materials sold in vacuum-packaging and sealed plastic pots with glossy labels and promoted by mighty marketing machines.

The wholefood movement suited my temperament at the time, and I still owe a debt of gratitude towards it. For one thing, the first article I ever wrote that reached printed status was written for a wholefood cookbook in the late 1970s. In it I argued that the practice of taking a perfectly formed and wholesome grain, stripping it of the parts that contained the greater proportion of its nutritional value—the husk (fibre) and the germ (vitamins)—leaving basically the endosperm (starch), was thinly disguised madness, especially given that many of the products—including bread and cereal—made from this remnant had to be "fortified" by having a small range of the nutrients industrially reinserted before they reached the supermarket shelves. Moreover, the refined endosperm itself became a health risk since there was now nothing left in the product that might attenuate the inevitable spike in blood sugar produced upon eating it.

The wholefood movement went in many cases hand in hand with vegetarianism, and a little later, veganism. Once again, there were distortions. The adoption of a vegetarian diet was as much reliant upon the animal rights movement as it was upon an ideology of health-promotion, and the two formed an alliance of convenience for many years, such that the carnivorous diet became associated with ill-health, and the vegetarian diet was promoted as ultimately health-promoting and somehow more "natural"—and definitely more "spiritual". It was nothing of the kind, of course. It was quite possible to live as a pallid, unhealthy and emotionally challenged vegetarian atheist, as it was to live a robust and vibrant life as a well-adjusted meat-eating meditator. It was never about the ideology, and everything about the simple everyday choices that were made in the business of shopping for food.

My own decision, upon leaving home at the age of eighteen, was to go vegetarian. I had long wanted to do so, cheered on by narratives that characterised the vegetarian diet as inherently more spiritual and thereby promising a more secure connection to some notion of universal truth. This idea largely owed itself to an idea of spirituality that did not emanate from my culture at all, but from the traditions of Asia and the Indian subcontinent. Nevertheless, it was an important move for me, engaged as I was in the business of redesigning myself according to values I had chosen, as opposed to ones I had inherited or been inculcated with.

A little later I became vegan, and this too was important. For a start, abstinence from cow's milk dairy produce was an important move in curing myself of the hay fever and asthma that had plagued the first three decades of my life. With the benefit of the perspective of years and further learning, I am now more inclined to the view that the decision to quit *conventional* dairy produce was both wise and healthy—more of this a little later.

In these pages I am deliberately avoiding engaging with a value-orientated argument in favour of any specific food ideology. I am concerned only with outlining a coherent strategy for choosing food—whichever preference you have in terms of meat or non-meat, dairy or non-dairy, vegan, lacto-ovo-vegetarian, plant-based, pescetarian, paleo, keto, low-FODMAPs, gluten-free, dairy-free, sugar-free, raw food, macrobiotic, fruitarianism, or any other eating plan designed to deliver health. I may be passing the buck; but I am not keen to become a part of what I see to be the *problem* with food and eating in our age, which is the bewildering array of competing food and dietary *shoulds* and *should-nots*. This is not to say that any of the above-mentioned plans cannot be a serviceable intervention, with professional advice, in any specific health-related solution.

It is merely to introduce the two most basic considerations relating to food, *generally*:

1. Is it really food? Is the starting material presented in as original a form as nature intended it to be? Check it out by reference to what I call the "3 Ps":
   - Provenance: where does it come from?
   - Purity: how close is it to the original substance generated by Nature?
   - Processing: what's happened to it since it was originally harvested?
2. Before you start on blaming specific foods for your ill-health, have you also considered that the way you eat, and the fitness-for-purpose of your own digestive system, might have something to do with your ability to tolerate and benefit from food?

The second point we will address in the next section in this chapter. The first point is well made here and leads to the following guide to choosing foods that are clean, unadulterated, unprocessed (as far as possible), and yes, *natural*, in the sense of issuing entirely from the natural world without undue intermediary processing.

The one glaring difference between the way people tend to cook and eat in the current era, and the way, for example, I remember my grandmothers cooking when I was a child, is that that generation never had the 'convenience' of ripping open a pack of something, placing it in the microwave and waiting only a matter of minutes before it was (supposedly) ready to eat. Even my parents, both of whom cooked, and who never owned a microwave (at least not while I lived with them), were "spoilt" to some extent by a wave of convenience options hitting the market—why bother to peel, boil, mash and butter potatoes when you can snip the top off a foil sachet, empty its bland contents into a bowl, add boiling water and you're done? Why chop, spice and cook meat and vegetables for a curry when you can rehydrate the contents of a foil-pack in a fraction of the time?

Some will point out that cooking itself is processing. Yes, and the culinary arts are indeed as old as the hills. Where do we draw the line between "processing" that benefits us and that which does not? The answer is contained in the phrase "starting materials": if your idea of cooking is removing the packaging and inserting directly into oven or microwave, then there are a few steps that you have missed out.

Do you know where the ingredients that you cook originated? If vegetable in origin, how were they grown? How stored and transported? How preserved or processed? If animal in origin, how were those animals reared? What was their quality of life? Were they "treated" with chemical drugs and hormones to increase their yield?

I am always relieved when I get patients in front of me who say things like, "I always cook from scratch: I like to know where the food comes from, and if anyone is going to process it, it will be me." At that point I know I am dealing with someone who is at least roughly "on the page" with my ideas about food and eating, and it matters less whether they are carnivorous or "plant based". Organically—and preferably locally—grown fruits and vegetables are essentials; and, if you do eat meat, naturally reared, grass-fed, free-range and ethically slaughtered are the *sine qua non* of a healthy approach to eating those foods.

Supplements

There are arguments for and against nutritional supplements. You have had a taste of my unapologetically radical views in the Dr Christopher story in Chapter 1. I do not mind if you want to take supplements *as long as you have done due diligence in researching the manufacturers' methods and ethics*[2]. At the risk of being accused of condescension, I might even offer the opinion that if you *believe* that they are helping you then they may well help you—placebo, after all, is a powerful principle. But I am not even saying that their benefits begin and end with placebo: there is little doubt, for example, from my clinical observation, that magnesium supplementation can help to relax someone who is tense, and possibly improve their sleep.

My argument is twofold: on the one hand, the magnesium is offered on the basis that the inability to relax owes itself to a deficiency of this particular mineral, when it is as likely that the inability to relax has *caused* a magnesium deficiency, through placing an excessive demand on available mineral stores. The practice of supplementation rarely asks what causes the problem in the first place: it simply puts a band-aid on the perceived injury.

In the second place, when magnesium is in fact a plentiful mineral in the world of natural foods (anything green is loaded with the stuff), why are we finding it necessary to present the nutrient as a refined, drug-like substance? In fact there are legitimate questions as to whether synthetic vitamins and nutrients are truly equivalent to those derived from the natural world.[3]

In the midst of all these debates, Natural Healing first advocates that we commit to a process of "joined-up thinking". The conclusion and decision as to what path to choose rests entirely with you, but have you thought it through completely and honestly? Do you accept "supplementation" as a temporary solution to a perceived deficit, or do you view it as a valid lifestyle choice? Again, I am not giving you the answer to this, no matter that I might have made my own position very clear. I like to feel I am open to persuasion and will happily listen to any counterargument. That way I can test—and potentially strengthen—my own perspective.

For example, one argument for nutrient supplementation is that our food production and agricultural practices have so impoverished the soil that the regular foods that we eat contain only around 40% of the nutrients that we might expect to find in them. Therefore, supplementation is necessary to maintain sufficiency of vital nutrients and thus prevent illness and declining health. My response to this is, OK I can see how that might work, but surely it points to a few other solutions too, doesn't it? Here are a few:

1. Buy from local producers who are committed to the highest standards of sustainability. In my locality there are a range of local growers with smallholdings who sell their produce at the local Farmer's Market every Sunday. Some of them do not have organic certification—mainly on account of the cost of getting Soil Association approval, which they would rather save and spend the money instead upon improving their service—but if you talk to them, you will be left in no doubt about their commitment to organic and sustainable food production. The quality of their produce speaks for itself. It is not homogenous in size and colour; it can be quirky, twisted, bulbous, individual, but it is larger than life—and delicious. The first time I set eyes on a bunch of freshly harvested celery at one of these stalls my eyes literally boggled at the difference between the colossal thrusting, burgeoning spray of vivid greenery, and the pale, thin stalks that offered themselves as "celery" in the supermarkets where, sadly at a certain point, I had become accustomed to shopping.
2. Grow as much of your own food as possible yourself. Find out about organic and biodynamic growing, how to enrich soil by recycling

organic products (composting) and adding mineral content. Plants are the primary link in the food chain. They are there precisely to transmute the vital "chemicals" of the earth—minerals—and render them usable to organic life—including us. That's what they do. Learn how to help them do that better. You may find that your early attempts to grow food are distinctly underwhelming: a few scrawny tomatoes, a clutch of dwarf-like and diminutive courgettes; but persevere, get to know the plants and what they like, and you will be rewarded tenfold—a hundred-fold—in the fullness of time.
3. Support other local grassroots initiatives, such as *Crops not Shops*, which is a sustainability initiative that also aspires towards social change on the basis of reconnecting individuals and communities with Nature, through community food growing, land-based education, and community outreach programmes for vulnerable people.[4]

The more people signing up to initiatives such as these, the fewer there will be shopping the usual way and supporting the corporate, globalist economic hegemony. Make no mistake, if you are politically minded about food (and frankly we all should be), these practices are vital acts of resistance. We are, faster than many realise, entering the era of global corporate domination and engulfment of the entire planetary food supply, extending to: control of seed banks; the almost universal use of agrochemicals that have been proven over and over to cause serious health conditions, including cancer; blanket and unavoidable genetic modification with profoundly worrying unforeseen consequences; the "fortification" of foods with insect "protein" and other undesirable adjuvants; the buying up of ever-larger swathes of arable land by corporations whose agenda is definitely NOT the health and resilience of the populations of the world, and for most of whom, once you trace the money back, it leads resolutely to the same collection of billionaire so-called philanthropists—the same people who are promoting mandatory vaccinations, stratospheric aerosol injection and geoengineering, thought control and agenda manipulation via their stranglehold on the mainstream media, and the routine cancelling via social media channels of anyone who is "off-narrative", or with a semblance of a mind of his or her own. Forgive my cynicism, but these are not people to whom I would willingly entrust the basic necessity of producing wholesome and life-enhancing food.

It comes down to a very simple message: eat FOOD. It is then for you to decide what your definition of food is.

Optimising the fire of digestion

In Ayurveda, digestion is likened to a fire: they call it *agni*, or *jatharagni*. When it burns brightly, our power to digest food is strong. So much so that (despite everything I have said in the previous section) even if we eat bad food we can still derive sustenance from it. On the other hand, if the fire of digestion burns low, even the best of foods may turn to poison inside us. This is as close to a description of autointoxication as I have come across. In Ayurveda deficient *agni* is a direct cause of something called *ama*, which may be defined as "that which can be neither assimilated nor eliminated". Ama is disease-causing substance, and in Ayurvedic teaching is to be found at cause in most chronic degenerative health conditions. It equates in both Chinese and Western traditional terms to *phlegm* (also thought of as the product of digestive deficiency) and stagnation: a sort of malign gunk, produced in-house, that disrupts and undermines health on a fundamental basis. Dr Christopher called it "mucus"—after the German natural hygienist Arnold Ehret, whose "mucusless diet" Christopher also advocated.

Pollan's second injunction, after "eat food", is "not too much". Harvey and Marilyn Diamond (*Fit for Life*) also stress heavily the importance of not over-eating. It is easy to see why. Digestive secretions are not inexhaustible—and in some with "weak" digestion they may occasionally be further limited. Once you have "run out" of stomach acid and pepsin, bile from liver and gall bladder, and pancreatic juices, anything more you introduce into your digestive tract will not be processed and will therefore potentially become a cause of putrefaction, fermentation, and the retention of materials surplus to requirements.

The habit of overeating is endemic and has been identified as a major cause of inflammation throughout the body, most notably in the case of autoimmunity. Functional Medicine research has also confirmed what naturopaths have known for over a hundred years (possibly far, far longer), that the gut is the foundation of the health of the whole organism.

When American herbalist Christopher Hobbs wrote a book about herbs for the digestion and liver he titled it *The Foundations of Health*.[5] The phrase, *"A Liver and Digestive Herbal"* was added as subtitle. The book gives instruction in the use of herbs to induce and maintain a healthy digestive process, by looking after the organs of secretion and ensuring that they are equal to the task, and by actively promoting a healthy flow of the secretory products needed for complete digestion.

Two important hormones feature in the management of digestion, and both are vital communications from within. They are *ghrelin* and *leptin*, both initially triggered and regulated by the hypothalamus, but produced in the stomach. Ghrelin is the hunger hormone, signalling when the body is in need of nutriment. Leptin is the so-called satiety hormone, and it switches off hunger—so much so that abnormally high levels of the hormone have been described as *anorexigenic*.

Not many of us, excepting those with full-blown eating disorders, have difficulty knowing when we are hungry. When it comes to the "off" switch, however, not many of us appear to know how it operates, and overeating is endemic, often fuelled by such well-known and well-intentioned exhortations to finish everything on our plate (even if we did not load the plate ourselves) and to remember the "starving millions" of the world.

At primary school I remember that we were not allowed to leave the table until we had finished the food we had been served. One day, after having had my plate loaded with something particularly revolting involving processed meat and slabs of lard-laden pastry, I point blank refused to eat any of it, and was duly kept back after everyone else had left. Resolute, I continued to sit there, until (probably because she had to clear and vacate the hall for the afternoon sports session) the dinner lady took pity on me and surreptitiously removed my plate. The point is that if you use punishment as a means of force-feeding children then there are likely to be consequences downline, and some of those will impact on health.

We are each responsible for the food we put into our bodies, and the quantities. Manfully struggling to finish everything long after you know you have had enough is not a sign of heroism: it is a sign of an eating disorder. For those who complain that this trivialises "real" eating disorders, think again. It may not be full-blown bulimia, but it is a damaging and pernicious habit that can be surprisingly difficult to break, and wilfully to eat more than you need is indeed a sign of a disturbed relationship with food. Just because you share it with 90% of the population does not make it normal; and it can be responsible for a plethora of related health problems down the track.

The problem is that we have forgotten how to eat mindfully. We eat while tapping away at our devices, while walking down the street, while in business meetings, while watching TV, while thinking about other things. All too often we miss the subtle communication contained in the release of leptin, and we continue to eat long after the signal to stop has been given—or sometimes we sort of get it, and then, looking down at our plate, we realise that we still have plenty left to "enjoy".

Psychotherapist Paul McKenna has a theory as to why this happens. He says our minds are so busy engaging with other business while we are eating that we forget to taste it properly and thus deprive ourselves of the reward of enjoyment of food.[6] Then when momentarily reminded of the deliciousness of food we continue to reach for more, but too late, the mind has already travelled back to the prior preoccupations, or forward on to something else.

If we eat mindfully, the moment of satiety becomes more intuitive: we pick up the signal, and we make the decision to stop—or at least if we continue then we do so in full consciousness of what we are doing to ourselves. The "trick" of mindful eating is well worth mastering; it takes some effort and diligence, but it is a primary health-preserving and health-enhancing skill, and I estimate that a good 50% of digestive problems could be solved very easily simply by adopting this practice. Here's how.

Mindful eating

1. Always eat in a calm, relaxed atmosphere, and NEVER when upset, busy or stressed out. To digest properly your parasympathetic nervous system ("Rest and Digest") needs to be engaged. If you are in sympathetic mode ("Fight or Flight") you will not be able to digest efficiently, if at all.
2. Chew all foods thoroughly. Digestion begins in the mouth where carbohydrates are predigested with salivary amylase. Breaking foods down into smaller particles is also crucial and lightens the burden on the stomach. Opinions vary as to how many times it is necessary to chew, between 20 times and 40 times. I go with 30, for good measure.
3. Keep it simple: do not eat too many different food types in one sitting. To do so may put too great a demand upon the available secretory resources. Food combining rules may be appropriate here (see below).
4. Do not dilute digestive juices by drinking too much with meals. A little water to clear the palate is fine but avoid washing food down with litres of fluids. Conversely, however, drinking around a half

pint of water 30 minutes before a meal can provide liver and pancreas with sufficient fluid with which to manufacture the secretions we need for digestion.
5. Do not eat too late at night or leave at least 3 hours between your last meal and retiring to bed. Once you are asleep no digestion will take place—or at least it will take place very slowly, and it may well disrupt your sleep. The optimal time for your main meal of the day is lunchtime, but this rarely suits our current cultural work patterns, so do what you can to eat early in the evening: 8pm should be the cut-off point.

Mindful eating is a practice, and like any other it demands commitment and development. It will reward you many times over, however, once you master it, with increased vitality, lowered inflammatory responses, reduced brain-fog, weight loss, and much more. It should be a fundamental component of any healing initiative.

A word in this context about social eating. You might think that because the attention is on the social interactions that this again divides it from the business of eating food. Indeed, in some meditative traditions eating is required routinely to be conducted in silence, sometimes to the extent of monks isolating specifically in order to eat. However, in my view social eating is something that is very natural and intuitive to human relationships, and so long as the social environment is not contentious, querulous or demanding, maintaining light-hearted conversation and sharing can enhance digestion. This is because when we are in that community sharing mode, we are far more likely to be in a heart-centred emotional and psychological space, which is very much an activator of the parasympathetic response—*rest and digest*—essential for efficient digestion to take place.

Food combining

Food combining, while originating as a weight-loss strategy, has at its heart the same values as those just discussed. It is successful in weight loss precisely because it enables and optimises digestion. Around the time I started practising, the Hay Diet was regaining popularity, having originally been formulated by William Howard Hay in the 1920s. It is essentially a naturopathic diet, having as a core principle the necessity to maintain a balance between acidity and alkalinity, and it was immensely influential on other researchers and practitioners downline, including Dr Robert O. Young,[7] and of course the Diamonds, whose *Fit for Life* we have already mentioned.

Some ideas, such as the need to separate proteins and carbohydrates in the same meal, go against currently accepted ideas, specifically in the management of blood sugar, where it is generally recognised that including protein *with* carbohydrate is essential for effective blood sugar management in diabetic and pre-diabetic patients. However, there is much of value in the system as a whole. The distilled rules of food combining are as follows:

1. Eat only lightly at breakfast. Overnight your cells put out their "trash" into the extracellular matrix for collection by the lymph system, which as we have seen then conveys it to the organs of elimination. First thing in the morning your system is still clearing out the residues of the day before. Fruit is ideal, as it is high water content and invigorating owing to the natural sugars contained.[8] Fruits, however, are very easily and quickly digested and should be consumed alone or before meals, as they may be held up in the digestive tract and start to ferment.
2. Your main meal of the day should be lunch, or after 12pm. In Ayurveda the fire of digestion is considered to burn most brightly during full daylight hours, and on that account this is the time to eat the bulk of concentrated foods. Ideally allow time for digestion to take place: there is a clear tendency for people to want to fall asleep after lunch, and while minimising carbohydrate intake can offset this to some degree, it may also be the case that this is natural economy at work: it means that the system is able to devote all its resources to the all-important function of digestion. In many Mediterranean countries you can still find the custom of resting after lunch throughout the early afternoon, the hottest part of the day—the *siesta*.
3. Do not drink too much with meals, for fear of diluting the all-important digestive secretions, especially the stomach acid.
4. Your final meal of the day should be as early as possible (8pm at the latest but preferably earlier), and again, it should be relatively light. A period of at least three hours should be allowed to elapse between your final meal and retiring to bed.

This is not an easy programme to stick to. We have not organised our economy around these rules at all, and we allow at best a perfunctory lunch period sandwiched between two monolithic slabs of work. So torpid are we in the afternoon that we often need to be revived by caffeine and sugar at "teatime", only to plough on another two or three hours before taking the transport homeward to a late, and rather full, main meal. We fall asleep with this barely digested and wake in the morning feeling groggy and hung over. One of the reasons I went self-employed at the first opportunity was to allow myself the luxury of organising my day around my physiological needs, rather than around everyone else's fiscal needs. Even so, one can find oneself at odds with the world. No one else keeps these hours, so doing business can occasionally be hit and miss. Without strict determination it becomes all too behovely to sync in with the herd!

To be or not to be "Plant based"?

At the outset of this chapter, I declared that I would not get involved in value judgements about dietary choice, and one of the most fundamental ideological divisions in these terms in our current era is the carnivore versus vegetarian debate. The term "plant-based" is a classic example of the contemporary preference for conflict avoidance. A "plant-based" diet could be anything—and frequently is. It is not even necessarily vegetarian or vegan, since it leaves the way open to including other foods as long as the "base" of what you eat is derived from plants.

The "plant-based" food trend has given rise to some of the least healthy options available on our shop and supermarket shelves, predicated as they are on oils so highly heated they have virtually become plastics, and processing on a scale never before seen in food production—lightyears onward from margarine, the original "healthy fat" replacement for butter. In one notorious case a well-known UK food chain is marketing products containing insect protein as "plant-based". Sugar itself is a "plant-based" product, but enough has been written about its deleterious effects to make it unnecessary to repeat the warnings here.

Pollan's third injunction—"Mainly plants"—nonetheless reflects an important perspective. As previously noted, plants are primary requirements for all animal life (although since they themselves have been found to be reliant in turn upon fungi, we might soon find ourselves revising this belief[9]) and contain within them the potential to supply all our dietary needs without aggressive processing, which these days is often carried out to make them look and taste more like meat and dairy products. What Pollan means is that, whether or not we eat animal-derived foods, our diet should predominantly rely upon plants—not "plant-based" substances, but PLANTS.

Meat eaters often complain that a vegan diet must be "boring". But upon what do they base this assumption? There are literally hundreds, possibly thousands, of available food plants, which also cover the full range of seasonal expressions of plants—leaves, flowers, seeds, fruits, squashes, roots, rhizomes and stems. Among this extraordinary cornucopia the possible combinations are endless, especially if combined with culinary herbs and spices for flavouring.

I recently went to a very interesting "concept restaurant", where we were served around a dozen dishes from a "taster menu". The restaurant described their cuisine as "plant-led", and although not 100% vegan (they did use some milk products) was constructed exclusively in cooperation with high-quality local UK producers. I estimated that at the end of that "meal" I had probably consumed a greater number of different plants than I had during the entire previous decade! Diversity of plant consumption is in fact important, as it maximises the potential for provision of key micronutrients.

There are two health-related concerns about meat-eating. One is the far higher risk of parasite infestation. You can get parasites from a vegetarian diet, but it's far less likely. The other is that, in some constitutions, it can predispose to constipation. Many people upon changing to a vegetarian diet—or even to eating a higher volume of fruits and vegetables—gain instant benefit in increased frequency, completeness and comfort of bowel motions. Moreover, the consequence of maldigestion and retention of animal products in the digestive tract is putrefaction—not a nice situation. It is an interesting fact that carnivorous animals have much shorter digestive tracts: that stuff needs to be processed and expelled as quickly as possible. If you do consume animal-derived foods, I would counsel that regular bowel cleansing, and the conscientious avoidance of slow intestinal transit, is the minimum maintenance that you need to commit to.

Many vegetarians do of course eat milk products, and even eggs. That's the reason why the word "vegan" was introduced, to differentiate between those who simply did not eat the bodies of animals, from the ones who ate neither their bodies, nor their secretions, nor their nascent offspring. The "lacto-ovo-vegetarians" found themselves in an unenviable situation in the morality *and* the health stakes with some commentators advising that dairy consumption is specifically implicated in the aetiology of a range of chronic disease states, including some types of cancer, and type 2 diabetes.[10]

In the interests of balance, it may be necessary to point out that disease aetiology is multifactorial, and that the calculation of cultural and individual variables may cast a certain measure of reasonable doubt over such pronouncements. Not all people who drink milk develop breast cancer. Not all people who eat meat develop heart disease or colon cancer. Furthermore, there are incidences of locations in the world where longevity rates are high, with minimal incidence of chronic disease, yet where meat-eating and other supposedly "unhealthy" practices, such as the consumption of alcoholic beverages, are not eschewed. Such examples will be discussed further downline in this book, as we continue to explore the many factors that can contribute to a healthy and vital human existence.

In considering whether or not to eat animal produce, however, it is the issues attendant upon rearing, slaughtering and processing that we chiefly need to be aware of. Were I a meat eater, I would surely be choosing organic, grass-fed and humanely slaughtered as necessary conditions for purchasing meat. And as far as dairy products go, in India the cow is revered as sacred for the benefit she brings, and milk is an important food in that country, but there is the world of difference between the raw, natural food, and the commodified, homogenised, medicalised, pasteurised concoction, derived from enslaved and brutalised animals, that characterises the greater proportion of the dairy industry in the "developed" world.

As always in industrialised food production we are handing over the vital—and sacred—responsibility for the provision of food to individuals and corporations whose main focus is their own profits and those of their shareholders. In this equation the sentience of animals has no place and no consideration, and thereby Nature herself is diminished and disrespected.

Eat the rainbow

The colours of plant foods are important. They are signatures to the nutrients that the plants contain—green for chlorophyll, red, orange and yellow for carotenoids, red, blue and purple for anthocyanins. The colours, especially those in the darker regions of the spectrum, signal a high content of potent antioxidants. There are the micronutrients that we need in bulk alongside the macronutrients—proteins, carbohydrates and fats.

This is another reason why plant compounds (phytonutrients) should be uppermost in our diets. As we have seen, digestive processes themselves generate toxins, which then need to be buffered. Antioxidants are the buffers. Toxins very often wreak their havoc on our cells by "oxidising" the molecular structures within them. This means that they knock electrons out of orbit, thus destabilising the structure and creating "free radicals", electrons that can then proceed to destabilise nearby atoms and molecules in a chain reaction. The result is significant damage to tissues and organs.

Antioxidants "donate" electrons and thus work to contain and stabilise the situation. Nowhere is this more important than in the liver, where there is a huge need for the protective activity of antioxidants owing to detoxification processes that initially render toxins even more toxic. Plants, correctly chosen and eaten, can help to keep the liver optimised and protected throughout the detoxification cycle, and supply vital nutrients for these processes.

Chlorophyll is another amazing plant substance. The chlorophyll molecule closely resembles the haemoglobin molecule, except that at the centre of haemoglobin is an atom of iron, whereas in chlorophyll it is magnesium. This is why green foods contain so much magnesium. Our digestion is able to swap out the magnesium for the iron—also contained in high amounts in dark green leafy vegetables—and thus "build" blood for us.

However, we do not even have to think about all this "science": all we have to do is to ensure we "eat the rainbow" every day. There is something superbly elegant about a system that colour-codes foods naturally, so we are automatically guided to eat the right mix of micronutrients. It may also go hand in hand with the development of colour vision in humans and some mammals, such that we are able to perceive these effects.[11]

The question of how much of these foods we need every day is often catered for in the widely publicised advice to eat "5-a-day": the unit is a fist-sized serving. Some nutritionists believe 10-a-day is nearer to mark for achieving optimum health, although it has to be said this will challenge most people. In cases of chronic disease states, however, where there is a need to do extra work on this level, there is one method that can come to our aid, and that is juicing, which I will discuss below.

When assessing the diets of my patients, I quite often ask for additional information on this subject. Obviously, I want to know what they are eating but if someone tells me, "I had chicken and rice with vegetables", I don't really get a very detailed picture of what is on their plate. For a start the "vegetables" are not specified and appear almost as an afterthought. The strong likelihood is that the greater part of the meal (and considered the "important" part) is the chicken, and then rice, and lastly the vegetables—maybe a quarter or less of the total bulk. So then, I ask, give me an idea of how much of each food type is on your plate? That fills in some detail, but I still need to know one more thing: when you look at your plate, what do you see, in terms of colour? Are you, in fact, seeing that rainbow? Or, if not all at one sitting, do you include foods of all those colours in different sittings throughout the day?

As a rough guide, the minimum proportion of plant produce recommended at any mealtime is 50%. Your ability to digest the "concentrated" foods—proteins, carbohydrates and fats—will be further enhanced by combining in the mouth and in the digestive tract with these basic foods. This is because plants also contain important phytonutrients and enzymes that activate and support digestive processes. This is one key reason also for using herbs and spices: they are there for their taste benefits, certainly, but among the arcane secrets of taste are important chemical and energetic principles that act to perform their own miracles in toning and tuning the very mechanisms of absorption and assimilation upon which we so rely for optimal functioning across a range of physiological functions.

Juicing

Juicing could have been included in the chapter on detoxification, and in fact the twin pillars of detox and nourishment (cleansing and building) frequently overlap. One reason for this is, as has already been discussed, nutrients are needed to assist in detoxification, for example by optimising liver processes. It is the case that if we could live in a way that fully supports normal physiological functions the need for intensive protocols is reduced or eliminated. Detoxification is what becomes necessary when your natural in-house mechanisms are overwhelmed by what they encounter in your environment. Part of this is not within our power to withstand—it has been estimated, for example, that there now exists *precisely nowhere on the planet* that is guaranteed free from chemical contaminants. For this reason alone I suggest that detox is something we should all be doing routinely—as we will also see in Chapter 5.

The same can apply to juicing. I am often asked, why juice? Why not just eat the food? The answer is multifaceted and extends over: reduced nutrient profiles in foods; sub-optimal digestive processes; and stress, which can severely disrupt physiology, as well as generating its own toxins. It seems we need belt and braces in addressing our nutritional needs in this era, and juicing can be a way of maximising the nutrient potential of the foods we eat, by delivering them minus their cellulose packaging, in a form that can be quickly processed, absorbed and assimilated in the digestive tract.

When it comes to juicing, there is no real competition for fresh. This is because as soon as you break down the plant material and expose it to oxygen and light it will start to oxidise. Shop-bought juices then are arguably worse than useless—a good source of refined sugar, perhaps, and a temporary energy boost, but hardly a nutritionally sound product. The best of them, fresh-pressed and then immediately vacuum-sealed in an opaque container, may pass muster if you really don't have the time to create your own fresh and vibrant juices in-house.

The next question is, what type of juicer should I get? There is little doubt that the most expensive varieties, the so-called masticating juicers, such as the famous Champion,[12] are the best in terms of cracking the cell-walls in plant material and making available the full spectrum of nutrients for our use. However, if you are working with a restricted budget, get the one you can afford, and upgrade as and when it becomes possible.

Juicing is time-consuming and labour-intensive, so most people will not do it on a daily basis, but during detoxification periods it is an extremely beneficial adjunct to the protocols described in Chapter 3, and can, once you are used to spending longer and longer periods of time without "normal" foods, serve as the basis of a serious detox, even replacing solid foods for short periods.

Juice recipes are not hard to find, and you can also mix and match, devise your own blends and experiment. You can also think in terms of devising your juices specifically with the rainbow in mind. Here is an all-purpose blend for a tasty and fortifying vegetable juice:

- Carrot   40%
- Greens (spinach or fresh young nettle leaves)   20%
- Celery stalk   20%
- Beetroot   15%
- Lemon or lime   5%

  Add fresh ginger, cayenne pepper or garlic to taste

In general, it is wiser to separate fruits from vegetables, but lemons and limes can be added to any mix. If you want double fortification you can even use your juice as the base to make up the Blended Salad recipe described in Chapter 3. That way you get the fibre (adherents of smoothies often point out that juicing deprives you of the fibre in your food) as well as a blast of concentrated nutrients.

Cooked versus raw food

Some traditional medicine systems warn against using cold and watery (damp) foods where digestion is judged to be weak. As we have seen, digestion is likened to a fire, and it is argued that cold, damp foods effectively act to extinguish it. Therefore, oftentimes we are advised to cook foods in order to assist digestion. This is advice often heard in relation to the traditional Chinese diagnosis of *spleen qi deficiency*[13], and it has merit. Weak digestion, for example, may well not be able easily to break down cellulose, thus depriving us of the full benefit of nutritional principles derived from plants, especially, since this is necessary in order to access the contents of plant cells. If you suffer from spleen qi deficiency you will indeed be helped by eating foods that are both physically and energetically (see below) warm.

Against that we have the raw food lobby, which holds that cooking of any kind depletes foods of important nutrients, particularly enzymes. Raw food aficionados frequently argue against cooking as a solution to digestive deficiency by advising that food can be "energetically" warmed up using herbs and spices, and indeed it is true that pungent and warming principles in plants such as ginger, garlic, fennel seed, cinnamon and hot peppers do indeed act to stimulate digestive secretions.

The "answer" to this is probably going to be highly individual. Observe whether in either case your digestion is giving you signals of discomfort and adjust accordingly. Some do indeed feel they are unable to digest raw foods. If this is you, err on the side of caution and cook your foods with mild spices to enhance digestion. Happily, in most cases, we can combine and get the best of both worlds, which would seem to be the most sensible strategy, if in doubt. You also, however, have the possibility to improve upon your current digestive status with the correct treatment: for this consult a specialist—herbalist, nutritionist or naturopath.

Water of life

The final matter to consider in this chapter is fluid intake. Again, this has been controversial, with some maintaining that we need that all-important 2 litres of water daily to avoid dehydration, while others advise that we can get fluids through eating high water-content foods, and therefore do not need that much additional water. Need for water will also depend upon several variables, such as ambient temperature, dietary habits (predominance of dense and processed foods), alcohol consumption, and typical consumption of diuretic beverages such as coffee.

Before we tackle water in more depth, it is worth pointing out that as far as other beverages are concerned the same rules apply as have been cited in relation to food: think in terms of the 3Ps—Provenance, Purity and Processing. I will discuss physiologically stimulating or sedating habits such as caffeinated drinks, alcohol, as well as other so-called "recreational" substances, in Chapter 7, when we will focus on stress management.

Iranian medical doctor Fereydoon Batmanghelidj identified dehydration as an often-unrealised cause in a broad spectrum of diseases.[14] Working in a prison camp during the political upheaval in Iran, very few medications were available with which to treat his patients, which led to his discovery that simply ensuring sufficient water intake could have a profound impact on physical condition and diseased states.

In much of the developed world there is unfortunately a major concern over water quality. Read that again if you have to. We pride ourselves on having developed a universal water delivery system, which although it comes at a cost to consumers, is generally taken for granted everywhere in so-called "civilisation". As part of this, we are told, it is necessary to "treat" the water using toxic chemicals such as chlorine and fluoride. We may easily be able to understand the necessity for antisepsis and bacteriostasis, but there are substances in our regular water supply—fluoride itself is one of them—which have nothing to do with bacteriostasis. The fluoride story is well-covered elsewhere,[15] so suffice it to say that it is now fairly clear why we should not be ingesting it: from its carcinogenic properties to its supposed ability to contribute to calcification of the pineal gland, this is not a substance that has any business as a component of our water supply.

Defensive living

At this point I would like to introduce a key concept of this book: *defensive living*. I have referred to it obliquely in comments already made about food choices, and we will meet it again in the discussion on air quality in Chapter 5. What it points to is the necessity to guard very heavily the portals through which unwelcome elements may enter our domain, particularly the domain of our bodies. We all have a need for water, so we accept, and to some extent are justifiably grateful, that there are companies that concern themselves with supplying that vital commodity, so we don't have to trek back and forth to the water hole. But then we find out what they are introducing by stealth via that channel and those services begin to take on a more sinister aspect. At that point, although we are indebted still for the water, we need to find ways of screening out the pollutants and adulterants.

In a highly evolved civilisation defensive living should hardly be necessary—which begs the question, despite our overblown confidence in our achievements, how justified is the human race's assumption of superiority? Everywhere we stumble upon the evidence that for all our presumed evolutionary advantages, we are savagely disrupting the very fabric of our physical being, and that of our home, planet earth, with practices that are so highly toxic that it is unthinkable that any sane society would ever condone them.

In terms of water, defensive living entails the calculated removal of all such contaminants at the point of use. In terms of consumption, the only water I personally allow into drinks and cooking is distilled. If nothing else, once I had seen the blue–grey–pink, foul-smelling scum left on the inside of the distiller kettle after only one distillation, I was convinced that drinking water straight from the tap was no longer an option. Distillation is the only way to guarantee that your water contains nothing but H_2O, and distillers can be bought easily and these days quite inexpensively, although you do have to factor in the electricity cost of running them. In comparison to other options, however, such as complete in-house filtration including reverse osmosis, or buying mineral water, it is still competitive.

Filtration is the next best option, but even the most effective and microscopic filtration (reverse osmosis) will still leave some residues untouched to make their way into your bodies, in particular, bacterial microorganisms and dissolved gases, such as carbon dioxide, methane and radon. However, any filtration is better than none.

There are those who complain that because distilled water has no mineral content it will therefore leach minerals from your body. There are a couple of studies that suggest that mineral loss through urination is very slightly higher in those who drink distilled water, but the amounts are negligible, and if your diet is high in mineral-rich vegetables there is really no need for concern.

If you are not convinced by this then remineralising water is easy: make a *solé* by adding a thin layer of salt crystals (for these purposes use a whole salt, such as Celtic sea salt or Himalayan crystal salt, which contain a comprehensive range of minerals—up to 84 key elements in Himalayan salt) to the bottom of a 2-litre jug, then fill with water. Top up your glass, or water bottle, from this reservoir, and when the jug is empty simply add more water onto the salt crystals, which will very slowly disperse into the water over repeated fillings. In fact, remineralising with salt is also a great way to ensure your body is hydrated from the water you drink, especially in hot weather: remember that in the desert folk are advised to carry salt tablets in order to remain hydrated. This works because the body has to buffer salt to maintain the correct sodium–potassium ratio by retaining water.[16]

If you buy mineral water, ensure that it comes in glass bottles. There is a risk of leeching of chemicals into your water from plastic containers, including BPA (bisphenol A—a so-called "endocrine disrupter" implicated in dysfunctions of the female reproductive cycle, and a known risk to children, including those as yet unborn), heavy metals, and plastic itself in the form of nanoplastics that readily enter the blood stream, gaining access to cells, with effects as yet uncharted and unpredictable.

Defensive living is demanding, but highly necessary. It does involve hyper-vigilance in terms of the decisions we make about our exposure to a wide range of possible toxins. It is almost impossible, in a busy contemporary working life, to avoid buying the occasional meal out, ready-cooked or prepared ingredient. We just need to do the best we can—read the small print and avoid the obvious pitfalls. But it is also about remembering our routine detoxification practice, so that whatever we cannot avoid, or that which gets in through the back door of our busyness and inattention, can be successfully eliminated on a regular basis.

One way of becoming more familiar with your reactions and preferences regarding food is to keep a food diary for a period of a couple of weeks. You can find templates for these online. Here is a simple example of what that might look like. If you set it up as a word-processing document you can simply type as much detail as you need to into the grid. I recommend not changing your current diet before doing this, as that way you can assess the impact of your current diet on your energy and health patterns.

Day	Breakfast	Lunch	Dinner	Snacks	Energy levels	Symptom severity
Monday						
Tuesday						
Wednesday						
Thursday						
Friday						
Saturday						
Sunday						

Figure 6. Sample food diary.

Finally, it may sound completely obvious and unnecessary to state, but if you find yourself repeatedly reacting to, or even just not doing so well on certain foods, then stop eating them. A good plan is to check yourself, your overall level of comfort, ease and vitality, about 30 minutes after a meal. If you feel sluggish and bloated, or experience aggravation of any typical symptoms, you may suspect that, for whatever reason, you are not dealing with that particular foodstuff well, and should at least temporarily desist from eating it. You can if you like check for allergies and intolerances, although these can and do change with the cycles of your health. And you can also take measures to optimise and upgrade your digestion.

Fasting

No chapter on food would be complete without some comment on abstaining from food. Fasting perhaps belongs in the detoxification chapters as much as it does here, but I am intrigued by the counterpoint between eating and not eating: it seems to me to be an intuitive pairing, and as we will see, fasting is not all about weight loss or detox, or in fact any health issue, but is a lifestyle choice of its own for reasons that arguably belong more to our spiritual and mental welfare than to a strictly physical healing.

It is not within the remit of this book to provide a comprehensive guide to fasting: the reader is encouraged to research the matter for him or herself, and to seek suitable experienced professional advice in order to arrive at an individually appropriate programme. However, the advantages of fasting are many and profound, and include benefits to blood sugar metabolism, weight loss, cardiovascular health, chronic inflammation, cognitive function, energy levels and more. By resting the digestive functions the body is able to supply more energy to other important physiological processes such as self-cleansing, repair and regeneration. Fasting can act to "reset" the whole system.

There are many types and levels of fast, beginning perhaps with *intermittent fasting*, where for 3–5 days a week you ensure a gap of between 12 and 16 hours between the last meal of the day and the first meal of the following day. This enables the body to instigate deeper levels of self-cleansing, promoting ketosis and autophagy, whereby the body begins to burn its own fat reserves and recycle dead and worn-out cells and tissues. Then there are short fasts ranging from 1 to 5 days, and mono fasts where you can eat, but only *one* type of food—grapes, water melon or brown rice are well-known examples.

Longer fasts potentially require working up to by committing and habituating to shorter periods first, but can achieve huge healing benefits. Most fasts permit a certain amount of nutrition to be taken on in the form of liquids—juices, herbal teas and broths, or the "tree syrup fast" discussed in Chapter 3 as the kidney flush or "master cleanser"; however the most powerful will only permit water. Purportedly more powerful still is dry fasting, but this can carry higher level of risk owing to dehydration, and is not advised without expert supervision. In fact the more powerful the fast, the more important it is to do the appropriate preparation by gaining experience and familiarity with the shorter and easier methods first.

The specific advantage of the less demanding fasts, especially juice fasting, is that in most cases it will be possible to carry on with the everyday business of life. This is because juicing enables you to receive a basic level of nutrition, especially sugars, which act to maintain energy levels to a greater or lesser degree, according to the materials used. However, as Stephen Harrod Buhner notes in his excellent book, *The Fasting Path*,[17] it is only in the current era in the Europeanised world that fasting has been viewed predominantly as means of enhancing *physical* health.

This has to do with the culturally specific separation of body, mind and spirit that has been hardwired into our thinking for the past nearly 400 years[18]. Elsewhere, and in previous eras in European history, fasting was a method of retreat, aimed at strengthening contact with the sacred, and with our authentic selves. In that context it is perhaps not so desirable to bring the trappings of our mundane and secular lives with us into the fasting space. Added to this, as I repeatedly discuss, in this book and elsewhere, the engagement with our deeper purpose, and the work we need to do to develop our emotional and spiritual "bodies", will be powerfully curative to our physical existence, as all are one in the unified field of our lives and our vital energy.

Arguably the most important thing to know about fasting is how to end it. It is for this reason that, for whichever specific fast or method you use, you are advised to research it thoroughly before embarking, and to have the specific materials to hand for your re-entry into "normal" eating and drinking patterns. A fast badly broken, as I have discovered from painful personal experience, can be damaging and highly unpleasant. Get specific advice native to the type of fast you are attempting.

Our next chapter is about air quality—*Ambient Air*—and we are going to add substantially to the list of "non-natural" threats and risk factors. I do not bring these matters to your attention to depress you or make you feel inadequate and defenceless; but knowing where we stand is a good place from which to start making the best decisions for our continued health and vitality.

Endnotes

1. Campbell, P. (2022). *Eat Right, Lose Weight* (London: Lagom).
2. It is unfortunately the case that in the current epoch we need to be aware that a large proportion of the supplement and nutraceutical industry is now owned and controlled by the pharmaceutical industry: draw your own conclusions about the possible impact of this.

3. A cogent discussion on this subject can be found in Doug Boyd's 1976 book *Rolling Thunder* (London: Bantam Doubleday Dell).
4. https://www.cropsnotshops.co.uk.
5. Hobbs, C. (1992). *The Foundations of Health: A Liver and Digestive Herbal* (Capitola: Botanica Press).
6. McKenna, P. (2007). *I Can Make You Thin* (London: Bantam Press).
7. Young, Robert O. (2009). *The pH Miracle* (London: Piatkus).
8. These days fruit gets a bad rap in some nutritional texts, including Robert Young, as being acidifying and predisposing to diabetes and cancer. This view has now been superseded—read this study for a more balanced verdict: https://www.bmj.com/content/347/bmj.f5001.abstract Learning how and when to eat fruit is important.
9. See Sheldrake, M. (2023). *Entangled Life: How Fungi Make Our Worlds* (London: Bodley Head).
10. Campbell, T.C. & Campbell, T. (2017). *The China Study: Revised and Expanded Edition* (Dallas: BenBella Books).
11. For a fascinating account of the science behind this read: https://www.eyenews.uk.com/education/trainees/post/a-brief-history-of-colour-vision.
12. https://www.juicers.co.uk/brands/champion/.
13. In TCM "spleen" is related to the digestive processes of transformation, absorption and distribution of nutrients. Qi is energy, so spleen qi deficiency = shortfall of available energy for digestion.
14. Batmanghelidj, F. (2008). *Your Body's Many Cries for Water* (Falls Church: Global Health Solutions).
15. Read Bryson, C. (2006). *The Fluoride Deception* (New York: Seven Stories Press).
16. For more on this read Hendel, B. & Ferreira, P. (2003) *Water & Salt: The Essence of Life* (Roseburg, OR: Natural Resources Inc.).
17. Harrod Buhner, S. (2003). *The Fasting Path: The Way to Spiritual, Physical, and Emotional Enlightenment* (New York: Avery).
18. This separation of mind and soul from body is usually blamed on the French Renaissance thinker Rene Descartes, who famously pronounced, "I think, therefore I am", and thus drew a distinction between "the world" that was observed, and the observing principle—the "I". Arguments against "vitalism", the notion that the world, including our bodies, is a living construct, persist in Western science to this day, despite the powerful evidence that is beginning to arise from contemporary physics.

CHAPTER FIVE

Ambient air and the electromagnetic soup

No, it's not a band name—but it would make a good one for an ecologically aware act! When the term "ambient air" was coined in relation to the six non-naturals, there can have been little idea of the state of affairs that would arise in the fulness of time. This chapter deals with the most obvious, but possibly least regarded aspect of our milieu, or environment. We take the air that we breathe for granted: and thus, potentially, we are placed at the greatest risk.

We have little choice but to breathe the air immediately around us. We can practise defensive living with water and food, but with air, unless we live in an eco-bubble, like the character Mike Monroe, the environmental activist in the American comedy TV series *Northern Exposure*, we have little choice but to breathe what is immediately available. Mike's multiple chemical sensitivities drove him into the wild, but even there he was not safe and so he constructed a dome, designed to maintain a fully regulated, filtered, protected environment from which he rarely ever emerged.

Mike's dome, however, would still not be effective in defending against one of the unseen threats to be discussed in this chapter, that of electromagnetic frequencies, or EMFs, which now envelop us in most locations around the globe (maybe think about that the next time

94   NATURAL HEALING

you are cursing the absence of a cell phone signal!), and which penetrate solid matter to reach us pretty much wherever we are, unless we have a lead-lined room or a Faraday cage handy. There are, I believe, answers to all these issues, but first we must become aware that they are indeed issues.

In this chapter we will cover the issues of air pollution from multiple sources, but we will end by checking in on another naturopathic practice that can have positive health-enhancing effects—that of sun and air-bathing. Again, there is controversy at the heart of it: at the same time as being lured into beach holidays by the barrage of seasonal advertising and cheap deals (usually just after Christmas—you got one spending spree out of the way, now here's the next), we are also warned of the dire consequences of exposure to the sun, and sold a multitude of chemical screening agents that, as we will see, potentially make the situation much worse.

The rabbit hole in the sky

In late 2021, at the height of the Covid-19 pandemic, billionaire philanthropist Bill Gates, having placed himself at the centre of the Covid-19 vaccination campaign, was reported to have announced his proposal to block out the sun as a way of combating climate change.[1] This was to be accomplished by filling the stratosphere with chemicals similar to those emitted in volcanic eruptions. Two years later, whether or not by "coincidence", in early 2023, the incidence of "vapour trails" left by high-flying aircraft increased dramatically and noticeably. This situation pertains to this day, with some days achieving full white-out status.

The relentless criss-crossing of trails, which then disperse and spread to form a widespread high-level haze, has become an almost daily phenomenon in my part of the world, but I also experienced it on holiday on a remote island in the north-eastern Aegean Sea recently, where I saw an aircraft make three passes over the same stretch of sky, leaving three parallel trails of an exact length, and visibly switching off whatever device was being used to create them once the required length had been achieved. Within the space of an hour that section of the sky had become a white blanket, startlingly regular in shape. Fortunately, the sun was at the time in another quarter of the sky, but in the days that followed the same effects succeeded in almost totally obscuring the sun by around three o'clock in the afternoon.

Awakening to the beauty of blue skies now comes with the dread of the first trail being seen—usually in the early afternoon, but occasionally well-advanced even first thing in the morning. Rarely is there a day when those blue skies persist for more than a few short hours. The World Meteorological Organization has even invented a new cloud type to explain them: *cirrus homogenitus*.

In the months that have elapsed since this all started I, together with many of the people who come to me for help, have experienced an unprecedented run of upper and lower respiratory tract complaints that have proved very difficult to resolve—at least without intervention. On "bad spray days" we also have a variety of additional symptoms—itchy, crawling skin, severe eye irritation, dry mouth and increased asthmatic wheezing in susceptible individuals—usually ascribed to "hay fever" and atopic allergies. The other explanation to which people resort is that we have all been adversely afflicted in the respiratory department since Covid—and this itself is by no means a baseless argument, of course.

I am not an expert in the precise technological parameters in such phenomena, and I have no wish to alienate my readers by presenting myself as a card-carrying member of the "tin foil hat" brigade. Talk of "chemtrails" typically brings accusations of promoting conspiracy theory and is an easy way to get cancelled. However, more and more people in my circle (which is a relatively large one given that I deal on a daily basis with the general public and their health concerns, and with hundreds of students) are noticing these effects and are concerned about them.

That notwithstanding, something has changed within this narrative in recent months. From being denounced as "conspiracy theory" for decades, it is now quite suddenly in the public domain, where reporting on geoengineering through SAI (stratospheric aerosol injection) and SRM (solar radiation management) initiatives has been seen in major mainstream media organs such as the BBC[2] and the *Guardian*[3] newspaper.

So why the change? Well, mainly, the emergence of an additional mainstream narrative that is being recruited to justify these practices: that of man-made climate change. Again, it is hardly my intention to enter this debate, or risk being dubbed "climate change denier": it would be the sheerest idiocy to deny that the climate is changing, and there is a sizeable chance that humans have a part to play in it. The open question is, by what mechanism? We are led to believe that is the burning of fossil fuels that is the problem, but it may be a whole lot more complicated than that.

We are now being sold a "solution" to the problem, consisting in this high-altitude experimentation, the consequences of which, research clearly indicates, are largely unknown—even in terms of the desired outcome—but expected among critical observers to be fairly catastrophic, with fallout (literally) affecting health, agriculture, weather patterns and eco-diversity. Could the proposed solution to the problem of global warming be as bad or potentially worse than the problem itself? Could it even contribute to the central problem? Putting a layer of stuff up at high altitude sounds an awful lot like creating a greenhouse to me: surely if you keep heat out of the system you also run the risk of keeping heat IN? But what do I know?

At the same time, the first few months of both 2023 and 2024 in the UK were uncommonly wet—and that's saying something, for the UK is characteristically damp at the best of times. The transition from 2023 to 2024 was almost unprecedented. I counted maybe ONE day on which it did not rain in over two months; and again, with the dampest of days, the dampest of symptoms—coughs, sneezes, sinus congestion, wheezes. Come May 2024 Brits were being told that this was the hottest summer on record, globally, while at the same time shivering in temperatures that barely rose above single figures and having to fire up the central heating at the precise season we'd usually be turning it off. Understandably, belief in global warming became for many a jarring cognitive dissonance and led to suspicions of gaslighting on a grand scale.

The other focus for these practices of course is weather-control (geoengineering), and this is accomplished not only by technology aimed at "cloud-seeding" but also, reportedly, by the introduction of HAARP—the High-frequency Active Auroral Research Program, which utilises high-frequency radio waves to excite the ionosphere, ostensibly in order to facilitate radio communications.

Although, predictably, scientists distance themselves from the accusation that this technology is deployed as a method of weather control, there are two questions that require answers: one, is the incidence of severe and extreme weather patterns coinciding with known HAARP activity (such as the recent flooding in Dubai) simply that—coincidence? Two, if you muck about with important components of the earth's atmosphere, is it not likely that you will end up influencing the weather? I might express the (inexpert) opinion that no realistic debate about climate change can take place without admitting the need to discuss these practices in context, which (and here is the cruncher) are NOT NEW. HAARP has been in operation since 1993, and stratospheric spreading goes back at least as far as the 1960s.[4]

I realise that I will be attracting a reputation throughout this book as someone who has scant regard for the official narratives in any direction, and for this I can scarcely apologise. But my business is health and assisting people to maintain and improve resilience and vitality across a variety of parameters, and in despite of multiple threats. In this endeavour I am necessarily acutely attuned to the effects that accrue from these aspects of our contemporary environment to the general level of health in our population, and to specific issues affecting respiratory health. You are perfectly entitled, and entirely welcome, to doubt and question my conclusions, but until you research it for yourself, as I have, I suggest you cannot knowledgeably denounce them. For myself, I remain open to dissuasion: these are not effects in which I *prefer* to believe.

In terms of what, exactly, we are being sprayed with, the one ingredient that has stood out not only to myself and other lay researchers, but also to mainstream observers and commentators such as the *British Medical Journal*, is aluminium.[5] Aluminium has been in the frame for some years now as a likely contributory cause of Alzheimer's Disease, the incidence of which, along with other neurocognitive pathologies, is approaching the proportions of an epidemic. Natural occurrence of atmospheric aluminium is associated with volcanic activity—upon which Gates's SRM strategy was reputedly modelled—and, according to the NIH (National Institute for Health) "the natural weathering of rocks"[6]—and although variable according to location, is a relatively stable, low-level phenomenon, with incidence reported to be in the range of 0.005 to 0.18 μg/m3.[7] Anthropogenic activity has already resulted in a significant increase in the levels of aluminium found in rainwater, with causation including industrial processes, fossil fuel emissions, waste incineration, mining, and "satellite demise"—the incidence of satellites falling out of orbit and burning up in the ozone layer.[8] These, it is suggested, are the primary causes, with SAI technology coming up rapidly on the inside lane.

If you want to know exactly what the aerosols are composed of, it is not difficult to discover, especially if you ditch Google and Yahoo and use search engines that allow you to access information largely hidden to the masses. There are literally hundreds of scientific papers available, such as the one cited here: but I did have to go via a different route to access them. Deruelle (2021) first makes mention of the theory that the behaviour of "genuine" aircraft trails will naturally vary according to atmospheric conditions, but then notes:

> ... other official documents link these persistent trails to a weather modification technology called solar geo-engineering by stratospheric aerosol injection (SAI). These sprays would be mainly composed of metallic particles (Al, Ba, Sr, Fe, nanoparticles) and sulfur, which would considerably increase air, soil and water pollution. Many of the current environmental and health problems are consistent with those described in the literature on solar geoengineering by SAI if this method was employed.[9]

The official narrative is that of course this is all speculative, no-one's actually doing any of it, it's all just an idea that has been proposed. Other sources suggest that it has indeed been going on for at least two decades and possibly far longer—probably on the basis that it would be difficult to recommend such technology to the government without experimental data to back it up, and the plain fact that it would be nigh-on impossible to provide such data until and unless someone did, actually, do it. And the problem with stuff up in the sky is, let's face it, it's difficult to hide, even from a population that has become inured to gaslighting on many fronts within recent history. Hence, perhaps, the sudden attempt to put a fancy frame around it: yes, it's happening, and yes, it might be a bit toxic, *but it's for your own good*.

Defensive strategies

What we are concerned with here, however, is what we can do about it. In the end, the question of what and who is responsible is one for which history will have to pass its verdict in the fulness of time. But the fact that it is happening, that air quality is declining fast all over the planet, is not in doubt, and that leaves us with a huge problem in terms of how we as individuals can respond defensively to it.

It is also the case that those most susceptible, unfortunate perhaps in being born with a high genetic risk for respiratory issues or compromised by previous affectations such as Covid-19, are likely to be in the front line of people suffering adverse consequences. For these people

Covid-19 and Long Covid are frequently cited as the most likely causative factors, potentially obscuring this additional insidious causation. Longer-term chronic pathologies, such as neurodegenerative diseases, including Alzheimer's, are assumed to be multifactorial, and we would need carefully constructed prospective and retrospective studies to prove conclusively that they are being significantly hastened and amplified by this relentless aerial bombardment of toxins. There is certainly data for pollution caused by fossil fuel combustion in urban environments: far fewer for what I plainly observe happening to clients of mine from rural populations where those effects are largely absent.

One thing is certain, unless we do construct that eco-bubble in which to live, we have little choice but to breathe in the air that surrounds us and to hope that we don't get too badly poisoned by it. One of the ironies about mask-wearing, considered in recent history an indispensable measure for preventing the spread of dangerous viruses, is that when it comes to filtering out pollution as we go about our daily business under our skies, it may well become a necessity. Even before Covid I knew cyclists who would not venture onto the streets of London without a mask to protect them from traffic fumes. How long before simply being in the open air, wherever you are, comes with similar risks?

In spite of the dire consequences that all this may suggest, I do not intend to depress anyone: far from it. I far prefer to see challenges such as those I have elaborated upon as opportunities for both general and specific system upgrades to the physiology of our bodies. My engagement with the alarming and sinister character of the matter is only to make the point that we are defenceless only as long as we do not know our enemy. Once we do, we are in a position to make our plans and evolve strategies.

My hope, therefore, is to empower you to counteract it. I hope part of the answer is already starting to become obvious: whatever enters our bodies eventually must pass through one particular organ: the liver. Detoxification generally, and liver detoxification especially, is a practice that I advise all readers to familiarise themselves with and perform at regular intervals: we will revisit it further down in this chapter. In additional to that, living as cleanly as possible will minimise the load on the organs of elimination—and that takes in everything we have so far discussed—so that unavoidable additional burdens are accorded the highest level of in-house defensive responses of which our immune systems are capable.

I would also recommend that you look into what homeopathy might be able to offer. This system of medicine has the significant benefit of being able to take something that is inherently toxic and turn it into a remedy for that precise ill, and there are remedies available that are made from toxic "chemtrail" constituents.

Care of the lungs is of the essence, as we have already signalled in Chapters 2 and 3. There are certainly facilities that can assist with enhancing oxygen status—hyperbaric oxygen tents, for example, and technologies such as Kaqun water.[10] These, while they may not directly address or strengthen lung capacity, can at least take the burden off those organs while they are treated, ensuring that cells and tissues do not suffer the effects of hypoxia.

Herbs are certainly among the forerunners in therapeutic responses to breathing difficulties and lung health, having effects such as the clearing of old mucus deposits from all respiratory passages, upper and lower; lubricating, disinfecting and rejuvenating the mucous membranes; stimulating the local circulation and thus improving the absorption of oxygen; improving the strength and vitality of the lungs, and with them, general immunity. There are several superstars in the running—here are a few:

- Elecampane root *(Inula helenium)*: expectorant, mucilaginous, antiseptic, immune-enhancing, slightly pungent herb (pungency stimulates circulation). This herb also has a content of inulin, which as well as helping to regulate blood sugar can provide prebiotic support to the intestinal microbiome, thus strengthening immunity in the gut as well.
- Echinacea herb and root *(Echinacea angustifolia, E. purpurea)*: global superstar immunomodulator, but regarded in traditional medicine as a "cooling alterative"—meaning it cleanses and revitalises lymph, leading to a reduction of mucus and a more effective flow of available immune capacity. An excellent partner to elecampane.
- Mullein flower or leaf *(Verbascum thapsus)*: these unmistakeable spikes of lemon-yellow flowers, reaching a height of 2 to 3 metres, and springing from a basal rosette of soft, green downy leaves, are a one-trick wonder for decongesting the upper and lower respiratory system. Mullein has been indispensable in the recent post-Covid years and has come to the rescue many times in cases where lung distress has resisted other methods and even other plants.

- Plantain leaf *(Plantago lanceolata, P. major)*: mucilaginous, mucotryptic (breaks up toughened mucus deposits), cooling lymphatic alterative (cleanser), expectorant and antiseptic. This plant has the benefit of being very easy to find in the UK, and is also effective against bacterial, plant and insect toxins—stings and bites.
- Marshmallow root *(Althaea officinalis)*: currently the favourite mucilaginous, mucous-membrane-protecting root out there (and the leaf is also good). Marshmallow recently took over from slippery elm, which had become over-harvested and endangered as a result of holding top position in demulcent, mucilaginous herbs. Works well in digestive, respiratory and urinary tracts to soothe and protect the mucus lining.
- Thyme leaf *(Thymus officinalis)*: possibly the best respiratory tract antiseptic with its content of thymol, used industrially in antiseptic products and effective over a wide range of bacterial pathogens. While bacteria are not regarded as primary causes of pathology, naturopathically speaking, controlling populations and cleaning up bacterial debris and toxins is an important job in cases of respiratory distress. Thyme is also an expectorant.
- Astragalus root *(Astragalus membranaceous)*: this herb is not a lung cleanser as such, but it does strengthen the lungs. In Chinese medicine it is a "qi" (energy) tonic, and it has a special affinity with the lungs, and with immunity. In Western herbal medicine terminology it is an adaptogen, and it makes a good partner with echinacea in strengthening and bolstering immunity.

If your favourite respiratory herb is not in this list, don't worry—there are probably literally hundreds of contenders: Nature is not limited when it comes to the healing properties of plants, and if you can't find one to do the job, another will surely jump in to take its place. The important thing is that, especially if you are susceptible, or on days when you are badly affected by symptoms, you take steps to protect and heal the lungs appropriately.

The installation of air filters and purifiers and dehumidifiers in the home would also seem to be intuitively wise. At least you have some measure of control over your environment in your own home, and again, if the lungs are your weakness, it would make sense to do everything possible to protect them.

Heavy metal detox

I have left this subject for this chapter as clearly it has relevance here. However, there is not much more to say about method that has not already been said in the detox chapters, especially Chapter 3. This is simply to add into the mix that the routines already discussed, especially the liver and the bowel cleanses, will themselves do a great job in detoxing from heavy metals alongside any other species of contaminants.

In herbal terms people often bring forward the ones that have seen the most press in recent times—cilantro (coriander), chlorella and sea moss—but there are many herbs that can assist in the process of removing heavy metals from the system, and when these are combined in programmes such as the ones mentioned in Chapter 3 these can be highly effective. The ingredients of the liver flush, for example, including garlic in the smoothie, and dandelion and burdock root in the detox tea, are extremely useful for this purpose, but many of the other herbs in the mix—red clover, nettle, cleavers, yellow dock—are also great allies in this endeavour.

My strong recommendation then is to perform a liver flush at frequent intervals if you are badly affected—once every 3 or 4 months is advised. An additional precaution is to ensure to take some fibre at the same time—marshmallow root, or psyllium husk maybe—in order to bind the toxins to prevent them being reabsorbed in the gut and ensure their safe passage out of the system.

Note I have not mentioned testing for heavy metal levels: this can be done if you want to target these substances in a more detailed manner, but there is a cost implication, and in most cases I do not find it necessary. The results, including lessening of symptoms and recovery of function, speak for themselves. In cases where, for example, immunity is impaired on an ongoing basis and does not seem to be able to recover, then specific testing may be performed.

The other herbal mix I want to mention is the Special Detox tea. I developed this formula, using the available scientific data at the time, to combat the phenomenon of vaccine-shedding affecting people living in close proximity to those who had consented to take the Covid-19 shots. I had many clients who complained that they had become ill when their partners or other family members were vaccinated, even though they themselves had refused the vaccine. The herbs chosen were specifically validated for their ability to break down the infamous "spike protein" that not only characterised the original pathogen (whatever that was—natural or man-made) but was also a component of the vaccines.

This mix proved very effective in reducing the malaise that these people experienced, but in addition we later used it with benefit in those who had been badly affected and unwell since taking the shots. These are the herbs in the formula:

- Pine needles *(Pinus sylvestris)*
- Wormwood herb *(Artemisia absinthium)*
- Orange peel *(Citrus aurantium)*
- Horsetail herb *(Equisetum arvense)*
- Fennel seed *(Foeniculum vulgare)*
- Dandelion leaf *(Taraxacum officinale)*
- Nettle leaf *(Urtica dioica)*

Horsetail, in particular, is of interest in view of the precise subject matter here, the removal of heavy metals: horsetail is very rich in silica, which is a substance used in homeopathy and homeopathic tissue salts to remove foreign objects, particularly metallic objects, from the tissues and cells. The best way to take it is as a hot infusion, 3 or 4 cups daily at times of need. Remember when infusing medicinal herbs to use twice the amount of herb that you would use for a standard beverage, and steep for at least 10 minutes.

The electromagnetic soup

This is another subject upon which a book may be written, and indeed has been. Dr Thomas Cowan, who achieved notoriety for his resistance to the Covid-19 narrative, has advanced the theory that what we think of as "viruses" are in fact the effects of cellular damage due to electromagnetic frequencies.[11] Beginning with the revelation that the coronavirus pandemic had its origin in Wuhan in the same week in 2019 that around 10,000 5G antennae were switched on in that city, Cowan goes on to propose that "contagion" and the notion of contagious diseases is a widely misunderstood phenomenon, and lends his support to a growing concern that the idea of a "virus" itself may be a misinterpretation of the facts.

Yet again we find ourselves in conspiracy territory. The major problem with airborne pathogens, toxins etc., whether nanoparticles, viruses or electromagnetic waves, is that we can't see them, and most of us have no access to the technology that is needed to verify them. We are therefore at the mercy of those whose job it is to tell us what's going on, and in light of the fact that their testimony is too often found to be tainted by self-interest, fear or simple greed, or is the programmed response of those who have been told what to say, it is difficult for anyone with their critical faculties intact to give them full credence.

Maybe if the UK government in 2021 had themselves acted in a manner that revealed that they were in any way worried for their personal safety amid the threat of a "deadly virus" we might be more inclined to trust them. As it was, we ended up wondering what they knew that we didn't, so insouciant and reckless their behaviour seemed, as they partied in Downing Street while the rest of us consented to isolation, including from our (sometimes dying) loved ones. Implicated in this scenario, unfortunately, are not only our governments and their advisors, but also the World Health Organization (WHO) and the National Institute for Health (NIH), two of the most prestigious organisations that purport to act on behalf of public health globally.

However, the debate on the deleterious effects of EMFs predates the pandemic by several decades and came into sharp focus in the 1990s with the widespread introduction of the first wave of mobile phones. "Excessive use" of mobile phones has been linked to: sleep problems, anxiety, digestive problems, dizziness and DNA damage including cancer. Many of these effects are due to the ability of EMFs to increase oxidative stress (free-radical damage), which disrupts cellular integrity by degrading molecular structure.

The argument set against these effects is frequently framed in terms of dose: the WHO declares that exposure to "low levels" of EMFs is safe: but what is a low level? And is this not also dependent upon the relative susceptibility of each individual? Any toxin you care to mention has two vital statistics: one, its own strength and virulence, and two, the resistance and vitality of the organism that falls prey to its effects.

The phenomenon of central sensitivity syndrome, or central sensitization syndrome (CSS), a condition closely related to chronic fatigue syndrome (CFS) and fibromyalgia syndrome (FMS), has been associated with this kind of hypersensitivity to environmental toxins, including chemicals and EMFs. The pathogenesis is usually via the mechanism of free-radical damage but is also thought to involve inflammation-mediated disruption of the blood/brain barrier, allowing neurotoxins to enter the cerebrospinal system.

This is important when we come to consider the role that plant medicines may have in protecting from these effects. But the point here is, that among those who continue to live and function "normally" in such conditions, the incidence of those who don't is relatively small. Could these individuals, however, be a contemporary equivalent of the coalmine canaries—the first to succumb to the toxic environment, but a warning to the rest of us, should the situation be allowed to continue and worsen?

There is a parallel here with nuclear radiation: when this strikes it is either, as in Hiroshima and Nagasaki, an act of war; or, in the case of Chernobyl, a catastrophic accident, but either way ordinary individuals have little defence against it. However, what we do know about these effects is that there is reason to believe that plants, once again, can come to the rescue.

In the wake of the Chernobyl disaster it was discovered that the use of Siberian ginseng (*Eleutherococcus senticosus*) could protect against the effects of radiation; and a cohort of studies have suggested that other "adaptogenic" plants, such as astragalus, schisandra, ashwagandha and gotu kola, could similarly protect against the adverse effects of radiotherapy used in oncology—and also, interestingly, the adverse effects of chemotherapy, whether radiologically active or not.[12] The actions of these herbs include antioxidant (they protect against free-radical damage) and metabolic enhancement. The exact way in which adaptogenic herbs accomplish their many salutary effects in the body is not fully understood, but they seem to strengthen and enhance resistance and resilience in the organism over a multiplicity of parameters.

Once again, it falls to each of us individually to ensure that we are informed and protected as far as possible. In the face of adversity of any kind it is the baseline of our health that will determine whether we overcome it or are overwhelmed by it. There is no essential difference in the advice given here than in any other part of this book: regular detoxification to ensure clear metabolic pathways, optimum nutrition to ensure a plentiful supply of the building blocks of a robust and resilient system, the use of health-enhancing practices such as hydrotherapy and movement, and above all, the specialised medicine of plants.

In respect of the specific toxicity of EMFs and other health-disrupting influences, there is a fair amount of talk about the mineral shungite. Shungite is a rare black stone that gets its name from the village of Shunga in Russia, where it was first identified. Its composition is 99% carbon, present in very specific molecular formations called *fullerenes*,

3-D spherical molecules made of 60 carbon atoms and having a hollow centre; but it also reportedly contains, in the other 1%, every other element in the periodic table.[13]

Among shungite's reputed benefits are antibacterial and antiviral properties, the ability to protect against oxidative damage, the ability to potentiate antioxidant enzymes, and the ability to purify water. You can also treat water with shungite: simply immerse the stone in a jug of water and let it do what it does, then drink the water. This practice has been credited with the ability to improve a wide range of symptoms, including allergies, autoimmune inflammation, viral or bacterial infections, digestive problems and chronic fatigue.

The sunshine of our lives?

There is one further topic to cover in this chapter on ambient air, and it is that of exposure to the sun. Once again, we are subject to conflicting narratives: sun exposure is necessary for the synthesis of vitamin D (true); but sun exposure is also a cause of skin damage including cancer. Once again, the matter of dose is paramount in determining the level of risk, but again, there is no clear advice on what a suitable dose is, with most conventional sources limiting it to 10–15 minutes daily. Once again, individual constitution is going to be major influence—if you are dark-skinned, for example, you are already adapted to spending longer periods in the sun without risk of harm, while fair skins are typically at greater risk of sunburn and the damage that accompanies it.

In naturopathic terms sun and air exposure is a salutary practice that enhances health in several ways, not merely by enhancing vitamin D synthesis; here are some:[14]

- Contains infrared, which has many benefits
- Contains full spectrum light, which increases dopamine and serotonin and can improve mitochondrial function (red light)
- Increases beta-endorphins, improving mood
- Relaxes the nervous system
- Increases nitric oxide, which helps improve blood flow
- Lowers inflammation
- Increases metabolism
- Is antimicrobial against fungi, bacteria, viruses, etc.
- Increases CD8 cells, which help the immune system

- Improves glutathione synthesis (an antioxidant responsible for its protective effects on tissues, especially the liver)
- Breaks down excess adrenaline, oestrogen, cortisol, prolactin, progesterone and testosterone

There are clearly reasons why we all feel better when the sun shines, and it is well-known that some individuals are especially sensitive to the reduction of sunlight in the winter months—seasonal affective disorder (SAD syndrome) is by no means a rare phenomenon in the UK, and involves a disruption of the serotonin–melotonin balance effected through the reception and transduction of light energy via the pineal gland.

We are however also frequently counselled to use "appropriate" protection against the sun in the form of chemical sunscreen preparations. These, as you may suspect, are problematic, and many of the chemicals used have been implicated in the aetiology of cancer, prompting the question, once again, as to whether the "cure" for sun-exposure may be worse than its ill-effects. As I have already noted in Chapter 2, to baste yourself in toxic chemicals and then lay yourself out in full sunlight to roast like a side of beef may be asking for trouble.

Once again, plants come to our rescue. If you need, or want, to spend lengthier periods of time in the sun, the following oils are effective in helping protect you:

- Jojoba oil (not strictly an oil, but a wax)—SPF 16
- Raspberry seed oil—SPF 25–50
- Carrot seed oil—SPF 35–40

I am not encouraging you to push the tolerance of your own system by using these plant oils to enable unwise behaviour. You must be the judge of how much exposure is right or beneficial for you. If you are paying attention you will not overdo it. If you are engaged in activities in the sunlight (and why not?) you may find these products useful to protect areas you cannot cover with clothing. Swimming, for example, is not an activity that one usually does fully clothed, and sun exposure during open-air swimming can be all the more potentially harmful because the coolness of the water may mask the strength of the solar radiation you are receiving, so it makes sense to oil-up before you go in the water.

Naturopathically speaking, we recommend sun- and air-bathing up to 30 minutes a day, not in the full midday and early afternoon heat, but mid-morning or late-afternoon, for the full range of the benefits listed above.

The air and sunlight is our natural milieu, or environment, no matter that we have developed a preference for houses and interiors. I would go so far as to say it is our birthright to feel safe and comfortable in the open air. It is not a freedom that I for one wish to give up without a fight.

Endnotes

1. https://www.forbes.com/sites/arielcohen/2021/01/11/bill-gates-backed-climate-solution-gains-traction-but-concerns-linger/.
2. http://news.bbc.co.uk/1/hi/technology/8338853.stm.
3. https://www.theguardian.com/environment/2022/dec/25/can-controversial-geoengineering-fix-climate-crisis.
4. Watzeck, J. R. (2021). *Climate as a weapon of War: H.A.A.R.P High Frequency Active Auroral Research Program.* Independently Published.
5. https://www.bmj.com/content/377/bmj.o1150/rr-1.
6. https://www.ncbi.nlm.nih.gov/pmc/articles/PMC8364537/.
7. https://www.atsdr.cdc.gov/toxprofiles/tp22-c2.pdf.
8. https://www.ncbi.nlm.nih.gov/pmc/articles/PMC8364537/.
9. Deruelle, F. (2021). Are Persistent Aircraft Trails a Threat to the Environment and to Health? *Reviews on Environmental Health*, 37(3): 407–421. Available at: https://doi.org/10.1515/reveh-2021-0060.
10. Kaqun water is described as "oxygen-rich, alkaline water", able to maintain a stable, high level of absorbable oxygen. https://www.kaqun.co.uk.
11. Cowan, T. & Fallon, S. (2020). *The Contagion Myth: Why Viruses (including "Coronavirus") Are Not the Cause of Disease* (Oxford: Blackwell).
12. Although there are many available scientific papers on this topic, it should be noted that the majority of these are based on rodent-model trials, which as Natural Healers we would distance ourselves from, but see Pang et al, 2022, https://journals.lww.com/md-journal/fulltext/2022/09090/efficacy_of_astragalus_in_the_treatment_of.66.aspx.
13. https://www.healthline.com/health/shungite#about-shungite.
14. https://health.selfdecode.com/blog/avoiding-sun-will-kill-14-proven-science-based-health-benefits-sun/.

CHAPTER SIX

Movement, rest, balance

This chapter will roll the categories of "exercise and rest", and "sleep and wakefulness", from our list of "non-naturals" in Chapter 1, into one discussion. A balance in work, rest and play is frequently advised in popular literature and standard advice-giving, but what does this mean? As always, individual personal disposition and character come into play. For one person, a holiday means time spent reading on the beach or walking in nature. For another it means sporting activities or pioneering excursions to far-off, and potentially slightly risky places.

Even in the matter of sleep, needs and habits vary widely among different individuals. Some will need their statutory 8 hours a night, while others will wake bouncing and refreshed after only 5 or 6 hours. Some will fare best with a nap in the afternoon to break the day, while for others this would be anathema, and an interruption with which they could scarcely cope in pursuit of their daily obligations. As always, not only individual constitution and preference apply, but also dose. Sleep is medicine: how much of it do you *need* to fulfil its natural purpose? This is up to you to determine, not for some all-wise health guru to dictate to you—and by the way, you can in fact have too much sleep: often those who silence the alarm and go back to sleep find that upon waking an hour or two later they are feeling more fatigued and sluggish than they might if they got up with their alarm.

In terms of work, not everyone wants to avoid it or break from it at the earliest opportunity. For me writing is work, but I enjoy it. I even sometimes take it on holiday! In fact, holidays themselves could be legitimately questioned on the basis that if your life is so arduous that all you can think about is getting away from it, then something is desperately out of balance. I enjoy going to different places, and actually working there. But if I don't know how to enjoy my life on a day-to-day basis, to make space for myself in the thick of the working week, then I probably don't know how to relax at all wherever I am, and there will be a distinct tendency to take all of that stress away with me. A lot of highly contentious arguments happen on holidays!

In our so-called civilisation we have the ludicrous situation where many of us put up with "jobs" we hate in order to pay the bills, while our lives slip by, scarcely allowing us time to do the things we love. If we are lucky enough to have jobs doing things we love, even for those of us who are self-employed, there is still the risk that market forces and global economics will intervene to cause us stress and upset that delicate work/rest/play balance.

Someone recently noted that the old hunter gatherers, far from having to work harder than any of us would ever want to, lived a life of leisure in comparison to the way we drive ourselves, and are driven, in our supposedly highly developed economy, where we spend our hours slaving for the wherewithal to buy the labour-saving and pleasure-giving devices that we never have time to enjoy. By comparison hanging out in forests and meadows waiting for the next rabbit to come along or sauntering over to the thicket to gather some berries, sounds like a heavenly existence compared with the life of toil that many are born for; and although admittedly there were still the natural predators to contend with, some might say we still have our predators, only now they wear suits and run banks. But then, the grass is always greener on the other side!

This chapter is about how to do the things that make you happy, and keep you healthy, in a balanced and effective way, and how to negotiate some of the obvious pitfalls in practice. It will be for you to decide what is appropriate for you and how you choose to implement the suggestions and advice given. As always in this book, the "advice" is usually a simple exhortation to think more clearly about the problem, apply the

Natural Healing Filter (or simply plain common-sense), and check in with yourself to intuit not THE answer, but YOUR answer.

I try to avoid the *shoulds* and the *shouldn'ts*. They are just another mechanism for keeping the grindstone going around. If you find yourself responding to any of the material in this book by saying things like, "I really *should* chew my food properly", or "I really *should* go to the gym", forget it. It's just another brick in the wall, to borrow a phrase from the famous Pink Floyd song. We are used to magisterial injunctions—it's how we were trained, most of us—but they rarely serve us well. We need to *want* to do stuff! We need to find the *passion* in living well, and in living naturally.

Moving your body

Exercise is a case in point. The very word is wrong. It comes from the same root as the word "exert", and exerting ourselves is sort of what we think we have to do, but there is something pedestrian and regimented about the ideas that are associated with this term. An "exercise" has the connotation of not quite being the real thing: it is something we may do in order to prepare for the real thing—whatever that may be. So we do it because we have to—because we *should*. If we have the sheer grit and determination to keep doing it for any meaningful length of time then all well and good, but for many people it's a short-lived resolution that caves in to the first temptation to miss a session, which then becomes the thin end of the wedge as we eventually fall off the wagon completely. I'm speaking personally of course.

I once attended a training workshop with a very skilful lady called Jan Fennell—the self-styled "dog listener".[1] Commenting on the way that wolves would conduct themselves in the wild, the civilised practice of "walking the dog" drew her satirical fire in all its comedic contempt. "Do you seriously imagine", she scoffed, "that the members of a wolf pack would wake up one day and say, come on guys, let's go for a walk!" Wolves in the wild move around for very specific, and life-preserving purposes: hunting, marking and defending territory, and migrating from one habitat to another to follow the available food supply. This isn't "exercise": it does demand physical stamina and agility, but it is purposeful and as serious as it gets. Little wonder that many domestic dogs have seemingly no idea how to behave on a "walk": for them it is potentially a life-or-death situation, fraught with danger, with risk lurking around every corner. For us it's "recreation". There's a serious mismatch in the way the two species relate to the idea.

Nonetheless, for humans, we should heartily thank our canine friends for their services in this regard, for without "walking the dog" some humans would get no "exercise" at all. That is to say, they would not move their bodies much further than reaching for the TV remote or going to the loo. That, by the way, is the observation of years in practice, not a lame attempt at a joke. There is something fundamentally lazy about humans. You wouldn't think so in respect of comments made above about how ludicrously hard we expect ourselves to work, and maybe it is a function of the hyperactive work ethic that when left "to our own devices" we frequently collapse into torpor and lassitude. We regard exercise as a chore, and in many cases that's exactly what it is.

If you are the kind of person who joyfully and energetically commits to an exercise regime, then I salute you. You may have a supreme evolutionary advantage over me. The capacity to enjoy routine, programmed exercise makes the job of staying healthy and agile, and developing stamina and endurance, so much easier. For many of us it's a sort of purgatory, and that indeed is often how I feel when I see people out running on the streets. Do they look as though they are enjoying themselves? Not really. Puffing and straining, red-faced and often on the point of flagging out completely, it is all I can do to stop myself from waylaying them and saying, "You do know you don't *have* to do this, don't you?"

The point I am at pains to make here is that, if you have found your preferred exercise type and are happy and satisfied that it works for you, then I am happy for you. If, however, you struggle with the whole concept of exercise, let alone the practice, then the following thoughts may help.

- What, if anything, *inspires* you to move your body? Is it a sport that you follow or enjoy? Team games like football really suit some people (less so others). Join a local club with players who are at your level.
- Dance: expressing yourself through creative movement is a practice that can be developed to a very high level of physical agility and fitness—or, if that kind of achievement is of no interest to you, it can serve as a fun way to explore and move your body, loosen your limbs and maintain flexibility. The enjoyment of music is an added bonus.

- If you are more of a loner, maybe running will suit you. Despite everything I said above, I used to run and enjoy it—just not dodging traffic and pedestrians out there in the concrete jungle, but in the country, on grass, earth or sand. On the other hand, I hated team games. At school I remember that I was offered an alternative to rugby in cross-country running. At first it was an excuse to stop off along the way with no teachers in sight and grab a crafty cigarette, but then my friend Nicolas and I decided for some reason that we might as well get something out of it and began to take it seriously. We ended up in the school cross-country running team competing with other schools—and winning (so much for hating team games!)
- Personally, having suffered a few accidents that put paid to my running career, my preferred activity these days is swimming. However, I can't tolerate chlorinated pools, which can be a problem unless you live near the coast (I do not). I enjoy wild swimming as and when I can access it, and there are opportunities if you look for them, although they generally involve some travel, and therefore are not everyday activities.
- What about activities like gardening, I am often asked? As long as we are not talking about the sedate Sunday afternoon deadheading of roses, I do think that a day spent taming Nature is a good challenge to the physical body. Horticulture, especially when put into service growing your own food, for example, as in cultivating an allotment, can serve the need for movement very satisfactorily, and has other very clear benefits—two birds, one stone. Later on in this chapter we will also meet the concept of *hormesis*—necessary and strength-building stress.
- Walking is probably the most intuitive and regular form of movement for humans. Walking wherever possible is a good way to keep your body basically fit for purpose, although unless you are a serious walker (mountain walking and hiking) it will probably not develop athleticism to any notable degree.
- Exercise classes: some people enjoy these …
- Join a gym. I have indeed purchased gym membership a few times in my life. Mostly it was a waste of money—although I always enjoyed the sauna and hydrotherapy spa. However, queueing for the use of resistance machines, weights and cross-trainers got very quickly boring—if only marginally more so than using the things.

- Hatha Yoga, Tai Chi, Pilates and Qi Gong. I have spent time with all of these and found them helpful, especially in rehabilitation after various mishaps involving broken bones and torn ligaments. I enjoy yoga the most, and having trained fairly intensively when I was in my 20s in B.K.S. Iyengar's style of yoga, I still to this day perform the asanas and vinyasas on a regular basis in the comfort of my own home (I do wish sometimes I had time to attend classes but for the most part this is a step too far in terms of logistics). It is a strong style, demanding attention, focus and stamina, and after even a short session I find myself refreshed and recalibrated, not to mention its value in the continued healing from my various musculoskeletal challenges.

To conclude, movement is both intuitive and vital. Your cardiovascular health, particularly, depends on it, and, as I have mentioned previously, your lymphatic circulation will not move unless you do, so it is also immune-enhancing and stagnation-reducing. It is well-publicised that those with chronic degenerative health conditions such as cardiovascular disease or type II diabetes benefit considerably, and in my work with people it is a base that we always cover, should the person not already be engaging with it. It is, however, best conducted in a meaningful context that offers other benefits, either practical, recreational or social.

One other perspective: in my previous book, *Practical Iridology*, I tackle the issue of exercise and movement from the basis of individual constitution as seen in the iris. Some types are well-constructed for vigorous aerobic exercise, others not so. Some definitely benefit more from core-strengthening—yoga, Pilates, free weights; others need to blow off steam and energy, and in fact have difficulty in relaxing unless they do so regularly. Find out your own type and plan your movement sessions accordingly.

The mother of yin tonics

This section is about sleep. In traditional Chinese medicine the term "yin" refers specifically to substance and nourishment. It is opposite and complementary to yang, which may be translated as force, energy and activity. The two principles are also regarded as the male and female principles, but the gendering of such concepts can be misleading—each of us is a blend of the two principles. In human physiology these ideas may be thought to correlate with the two major branches of the autonomic nervous system—the sympathetic (SNS –fight or flight) and the parasympathetic (PSNS—rest and digest). The point about these dualisms is not to prioritise one over the other, but to ensure an appropriate balance, and so it is with SNS and PSNS: they are equal and opposite, and we need both poles.

Sleep is then the counterpart of wakefulness. It is a necessary period of rest for the body, during which many vital functions are activated—detoxification, immunomodulation, reconstruction, regeneration and repair. This is why the Chinese dubbed sleep as "the mother of yin tonics". It allows the body the time and space to perform its self-regulating, parasympathetic functions.

For example, it is the case that specific immunity—that branch of our immunity that is responsible for synthesising antibodies in response to specific pathogens—is prioritised during sleep. It is even the case that when your specific immune system is engaged, as for example when you have a "cold", your body secretes biochemicals that make you feel tired and want to go to bed. This is so your specific immune system can get on with the job that needs doing. Conversely, during the day when we are active and alert, the non-specific (atopic) branch of our immune system takes over to ensure a baseline of protection. This kind of immunity is partly activated by rising cortisol levels in the morning, and so is associated with the sympathetic nervous system as it awakens to the challenges of the day.[2]

Insomnia, or sleep difficulties, are therefore in the long term a considerable threat to physical health and longevity, and one of the most important questions in interviewing patients will be to enquire about typical sleep habits. Here are some relevant questions to ask:

- Do you have difficulty going to sleep?
- Do you have difficulty staying asleep (i.e. do you wake during the night)?
- If you wake during the night, what time or times?
- Do you dream, if so how vividly, and do you get nightmares?
- Do you awaken refreshed in the morning?

I remember my GP (back in the days when I actually had one) telling me that difficulty going to sleep was due to "exogenous" anxiety—that is, anxiety about known things that keep one awake thinking; and waking during the night is due to "endogenous" anxiety—internal processes that perhaps are not normally in consciousness. Having often woken in the middle of the night and spent hours ruminating about troublesome events in my life I'd say this distinction is precarious. What I do know is that internal organ processes, especially relating to the liver and digestion, can indeed be responsible for restless sleep and waking at night. The Chinese, again, have an "organ clock" that allocates specific two-hour periods throughout the day to each of the twelve TCM organs. From this chart we can see that the nighttime is the domain of gall bladder (11pm–1am), liver (1am–3am), lungs (3am–5am), and large intestine (5am–7am). Of these slots the ones that most often arise in consultation are liver and lung, but particularly liver. I find liver therapy comes into its own very often in treating sleep disorders. One clue as to the possibility of liver-related sleep issues is that rarely indeed is it possible to cure the problem with the usual "hypnotic" herbs.

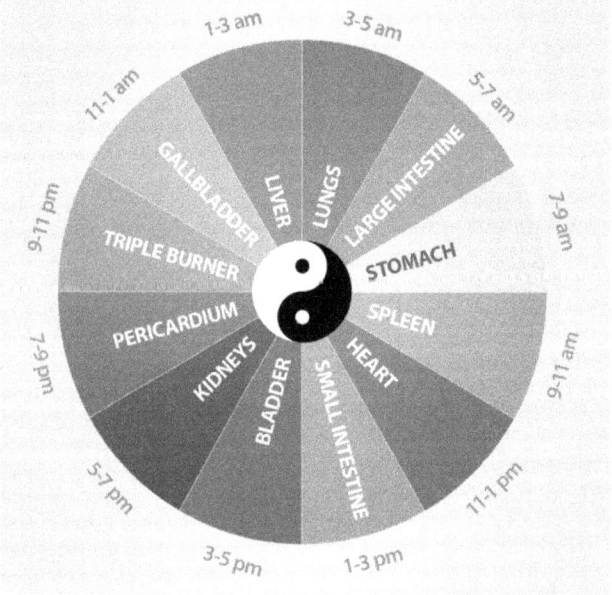

Figure 7. The traditional Chinese medicine organ clock.

Hypnotic herbs have nothing to do with hypnosis—they are sleep-inducers, but interestingly there are many cases of insomnia that do not respond to these powerful sedative herbs. Examples are valerian, hops, oatseed, passionflower and skullcap. If you get no relief from these herbs, then it is likely that your sleeplessness is due to an imbalance in another organ, oftentimes the liver: I have often found milk thistle to be effective in these cases, along with ongoing liver therapies, including the liver detoxification protocol discussed in Chapter 3. Abstaining from drinking alcohol in the evenings can also help.

If your sleeplessness does not conform to this pattern, however, there are two herbs that I most often work with: one is passionflower, the other ashwagandha. Very simply, passionflower is good for those who have trouble falling asleep, and is actually best taken as a bedtime tea, rather than tincture or a tablet (there's even a scientific clinical trial that specifically validates the use of the tea[3]).

Ashwagandha, on the other hand I have found most helpful where the subject tends to awaken in the small hours and cannot go back to sleep. The Latin name for ashwagandha is *Withania somnifera*: somnifera means, "bringer of sleep". As a light sleeper myself by nature, I have frequently resorted to ashwagandha when I intuit that my body needs a good, long, deep sleep. Making sure to take the herb only when I do not have to rise early in the morning (which I find spoils the effect and detracts from the feelings of warmth and comfort that the herb can impart), I freely take 3–5 capsules of the powdered herb before bedtime, or, my favourite way to take it, as a full teaspoon of the powder in a warm coconut milk drink. I will also on occasion combine both these herbs to good effect.

Simply knocking yourself out, however, without regard for what else may need adjusting in your life, is not a sustainable way to manage sleep issues—although there is always a place for a good sleepytime tea (see end of this section). If poor sleep is your habit, check into what may need adjusting: how is your "sleep hygiene"? Here are some suggestions:

Sleep hygiene

- Turn off all screens at least one hour before attempting to sleep.
- If you must use screens ensure you have a red filter installed on your device.
- A relaxing Epsom or magnesium salts bath can be helpful.

- Use an essential oil censor or diffuser in the bedroom and try different oils to see which benefits you the most. Relaxing essential oils include lavender, bergamot and clary sage.
- Try sprinkling a few drops of essential oil around your pillow—lavender is good for this.
- Try a lavender pillow, a small muslin bag filled with fresh or dried lavender flowers tucked underneath your pillow, or close to your head.
- Make sure your room is sufficiently darkened—use black-out blinds if necessary—or wear an eye mask.

Here is a herbal tea recipe that many have found effective taken about an hour before bed:

- Passionflower herb   2 parts
- Skullcap herb   1 part
- Lavender flowers   1 part
- Oat straw   1 part
- Chamomile flowers   1 part

Dreaming

Everybody dreams. I do occasionally interview someone who claims not to, however I believe we all do it but some, for some reason, do not remember their dreams. Dreams perform an important function for us. Dreams are where we often work things out that we cannot solve in waking life; where we process material that does not get dealt with completely as we go through the day; and potentially where we can access our own creativity in ways that are intuitive and perfectly aligned with our deeper purpose in life.

Dreamwork, the remembering and reviewing of dreams once awake, is a powerful means of self-discovery if correctly navigated—although I do not hold with stock-in-trade dream analysis: I believe the interpretations need to be guided by our own internal mythology and symbolism, not dictated by any externally derived theory. In short, dreaming is healthy and necessary—and by the way, it works whether or not you remember or analyse it. There is a lot else that could be said about this highly interesting subject, but again, there is plenty written about it elsewhere in both scientific and popular literature.

Vivid dreams, anxiety dreams and nightmares, however, may be signals of a potential problem. We are alerted to high levels of unacknowledged stress, retained trauma and an overheated mind. Very often they also point to heat and stagnation affecting, once again, the liver. The liver is very much a part of our stress-fighting machinery, which you can read about in my second iridology book, *The Mind's Eye*.[4] These symptoms are therefore useful in diagnosing sleep problems where they occur and will lead to the appropriate and relevant treatment responses.

Awakening

There are few things more aggravating, in my world, than being woken by an alarm. *Alarm* is the first stage in general adaptation syndrome (GAS) as described in the work of Hans Selye,[5] and it signals STRESS. There was once a time in my life when I had perfected the skill of setting my own internal alarm by means of pure suggestion and intention. As I got busier, however, one or two near-catastrophic failures had me capitulate to the inevitable solution. All I could do was to choose the least aggressive and jarring alarm tone from the iPhone menu.

Awakening naturally is a pure luxury in life. Do it as often as you can, especially if you find that you do not feel refreshed upon wakening. This symptom warns that you are approaching exhaustion (if indeed you have not already arrived at that state), and the last thing you need is to force the issue. I do realise that we all need to do what we must, and that waking up and getting up according to some timetable is largely unavoidable. I have certainly had my fair share of reluctance to awaken. My natural rhythm is to be an evening person—maybe because that's the time of day when I was born. There are those among us who habitually wake with the lark and are high-velocity from the moment they open their eyes. I have always been more of an owl, becoming more active as night draws on.

Whatever your preference and habit, note how you feel upon waking: are you ready for the day ahead? Are you dreading it? What would you do now if it were completely up to you? A leisurely breakfast? A yoga session? A walk?

There is one thing, however, that I strongly counsel you to avoid if you want to sleep soundly and awaken brightly: the TV, and especially the news. Since I gave up watching the *tell-lie-vision* my level of mental and emotional stability and equanimity has increased ten-fold. I now awaken to my own day, filled with the things I value and enjoy, including my work, as opposed to succumbing to the compulsion to join with the global madness and be by turns horrified, angered, sickened and depressed. Is that not a bit ostrich-like, you may ask? Well, bluntly, it's one thing to stick your head in the sand; quite another to fill your head with shit.

The subtle art of doing nothing

There is a time to be in motion, and a time to be at rest—not just at night during sleep, but being able to pace yourself during the day, to break up the performance of routine tasks and allow a shift of focus and a chance to engage your natural creativity. Writing, for example, is an intensive activity, and it is also a sedentary one. I have learned the hard way that not taking breaks may lead to stagnation, not just of the body, but of the mind, and a stagnant mind does not produce good work.

Far too often, however, we succumb to the notion that we must always be doing *something*. So, we can break from work, but we must do some stretching, make a cup of tea (OK if you sit down and drink it), write a shopping list, clean the kitchen, walk the dog, make the beds, empty the rubbish, wash the car, *open the emails* … that's the one that gets me! It's a fatal decision, that one.

Why not do nothing? Do we even know how to do nothing? There are a ton of injunctions against doing nothing: we might become a "good-for-nothing"; "nothing ventured nothing gained"; "The only thing necessary for evil to triumph is for good men to do nothing" (Edmund Burke). Or how about this one: "A life spent making mistakes is not only more honourable, but more useful than a life spent doing nothing" (George Bernard Shaw). It's alright, I do know I am quoting out of context, but that's the point: is there ever a context in which doing nothing is OK? I believe there is, both on the level of choosing not to intervene in every situation, and on that of resisting the compulsion to be engaged in some activity, however small, without feeling in the least bit guilty.

I recommend the following exercise:

- On at least two occasions in any ordinary day, put down what you are doing, sit or lie down, and do nothing for at least 10 minutes.

That's it. Practise to attain longer periods of doing nothing, until you can do a complete half day. More than that and life might start throwing you some unpleasant reminders, and I don't want to cause more stress than is necessary.

Watch cats. They are absolute masters of doing nothing. If you have a cat, it will probably sit on you and do nothing. Is that a subtle gambit, I have often wondered? Have you ever noticed how extremely reluctant one can be to have to dislodge a cat from your lap in order to get up and do something? You instinctively feel that the cat *knows* how good it is for you to do nothing together.

If we are being philosophical, we might say that *being* itself is never passive: the verb "to be" is an active verb. However, we rarely allow it to enter our awareness, and hence although we *exist*, the act of being is drowned out by the general noise of our lives, fuelled, in large part, by our busyness. Doing nothing potentially allows pure being to pervade both mind and body. This does not mean we do not think: it means that we are unconcerned with thinking. It means we need nothing, in the pure moment, but that which is there.

But the corollary is that doing nothing will inevitably give way quite naturally and organically to the desire to do something, not compulsively, but, if you are practising diligently, as an entirely spontaneous awakening of a creative impulse. Doing nothing is the necessary counterpoint to a life of meaningful activity. I am not talking about meditation by the way. That is different. I am a useless meditator; but I am very, very good at doing nothing. It is my first choice in accessing my creativity, and it reveals aspects of my experience that are impossible to attain through any other means.

Hormesis

Those of us who expect that life will proceed smoothly without incident or stress are probably fooling themselves. I am reminded of the gentleman who was interviewed on television news having witnessed a shooting in his street, wailing: "I'm just a normal man; I don't expect this in my life!" As we will see in the next chapter, no one can legislate for stress and traumatic events, although there are many things we can do to offset them once they have happened. Not all stress, however, is negative, and so we now come to the concept of *hormesis*.

Hormesis is the scientifically verified version of the quote, "That which does not kill me makes me stronger"—originally attributed to the German philosopher Friedrich Nietzsche. In other words, challenges are good for you. The theory is that exposure to a low level of stress or toxicity induces an adaptive beneficial effect in cells and organisms. A healthy body responds to mild stress by increasing its production of antioxidants and cellular quality control mechanisms.

Examples of how this can work are evident in calorie-restricted diets; the presence of plant chemicals in herbal medicines (many of which are actually slightly toxic, and yet can have obvious curative effects); exercise (the practice of "going for the burn", that is, taking things just beyond the limit of what is comfortable); cognitive stimulation (use the mind or lose the mind!); intermittent cold and heat (remember the alternating hot and cold shower treatments mentioned in Chapter 3). All these effects mildly stress the body, and they can all extend lifespan and health-span.

Nowhere is this more evident, perhaps, than in the so-called "bluezone" destinations of the world. The blue zones are relatively restricted areas where the inhabitants live longer than the average lifespan with fewer chronic diseases. There are officially six of them around the planet, and for the last few years I have spent short periods of time in one of these areas in particular. The island of Ikaria in the northern Aegean Sea is absolutely not known for its 5-star hotels, patrolled beaches with regimented lines of sunloungers, luxury spas, and all "mod-cons" accommodation. It is rugged, fairly original still (only relatively recently having gained an airport and a main road that connects one side of the island with the other), and still quite challenging to navigate if you want to get around the island and see what's there to see. Come October it gets distinctly cool, and though I have never been on the island in the winter months, I am assured that it is not the most clement of environments; and the locals work hard for their livelihoods.

That said, even these favoured localities are severely challenged in the context of the current global epidemic of "civilisation", and the tourist invasions that are one of the less savoury consequences. Once, people in Ikaria consumed food almost exclusively grown on the island, or taken from its seas, among which a daily intake of medicinal and culinary herbs often taken also as beverages. Now the bulk of food on the island is shipped in from Athens. Once they existed largely in the open air, their work practical, down to earth and conducted in the service of life-supporting industries such as food growing—both plant and animal—and fishing; now they perforce spend time in agency offices managing the increasing volume of tourists attracted by the Netflix "Blue Zone" docuseries and sundry in-flight magazines.

Their economy was turbo-boosted by the arrival of the airport in 1995, and there is now a fully metalled road that allows relatively stress-free access from one side of the island to the other. When my partner first visited the island in 1970 she and her then partner walked for two days over a 1000-metre ridge to access the southern coast of the island—and indeed walking was once the islanders' preferred method of transport.

However, their social life, where not disrupted by the necessity to import help from the city during the summer season, is vivacious, with the help of generous servings of very strong Ikarian red wine. Their social structure is evident to any foreigner entering the island: the "hardcore" islanders (where you can get to meet them) all pretty much know each other and look after each other, and they have a particular and special interest in their local culture, especially dance, in which they are known far and wide for the annual festival that takes place there. They swim regularly in the ocean, and many of them also routinely visit the many natural hot springs that are found around the coast of the island.

This strongly suggests that health and longevity does not take place in the context of a cosseted and protected environment and lifestyle. Our "civilised" preference for mechanisation, insurance, soft linings and soft landings is probably not going to result in the strongest, healthiest, most resilient and resourceful of populations.

My advice to you, then, is this. Spend as much time as reasonably possible outdoors in the company of plants, trees, streams, rivers and oceans, sun and wind, and the earth under your feet (take your shoes off!). Do your own chores. Eat wholesome, natural food, preferably grown by yourself, wherever possible. Exercise in a way that is natural and preferably in the open air. Do meaningful work as your contribution to the world you live in. Enjoy yourselves and each other, build strong relationships and strong communities.

We can, if we commit to it, create our own "blue zone" right where we are.

Endnotes

1. Fennell, J. (2002). *The Dog Listener: Learning the Language of Your Best Friend* (London: HarperCollins).

2. See Evans, P., Hucklebridge, F. & Clow, A. (2000). *Mind, Immunity and Health: The Science of Psychoneuroimmunology* (London: Free Association Books).
3. Ngan, A. & Conduit, R. (2011). A Double-blind, Placebo-controlled Investigation of the Effects of *Passiflora incarnata* (Passionflower) Herbal Tea on Subjective Sleep Quality. *Phytotherapy Research (PTR)*, 25(8): 1153–1159. doi:10.1002/ptr.3400.
4. Jackson-Main, P. (2024). *The Mind's Eye: Personality and Behaviour as Revealed in Quantum Iris Analysis* (London: Aeon).
5. Selye, H. (1956/1978). *The Stress of Life* (New York: McGraw-Hill).

CHAPTER SEVEN

Perturbations of the mind and spirit

In this chapter I want to talk a little more about stress. It is endemic to life on the physical plane of existence. Generally, we don't enjoy it, and we are endlessly creative about inventing ways to avoid it. Framing stressful events as inherently negative, however, compounds their power over us to disrupt and lay waste to our lives. It is entirely the case that occasionally something extremely bad happens to us—accidents, death, assault, divorce, theft and burglary, natural disasters and, of course, war—and I am not suggesting we deny how upset or damaged we are. In the midst of those effects, we need support, we need care, and we need to learn how to "detoxify" from the negativity that they engender, how to release the trauma and come to terms with what has happened.

But the majority of the "stress" that we experience is not on that level. You have probably heard the story of the farmer whose horse fell and broke its leg. The farmer had to "put it out of its misery". His neighbours all came around to commiserate: "How will you cope? What a disaster!" The farmer however remained calm and simply said, "Let's just wait and see." The next day a herd of mustang came driving through the valley, and his son was able to lasso and capture two stallions. Now the farmer had two horses. His neighbours were full of gossip: "You are so lucky! Yesterday you lost your horse, and today you have TWO horses!" Again, the farmer was unperturbed and simply said, "Let's just wait and see." The next day the farmer's son was out riding one of the horses when it bucked and threw him off, breaking his leg. The neighbours were predictably horrified and rushed round to offer their sympathies: "How will you manage now that your son is out of action?" The farmer (you guessed it) simply said, "Let's just wait and see." The following day the army came around recruiting young men for the war: the farmer's son was not chosen, owing to his broken leg.

I have a few times found myself rejected by people I was working for or with—in other words I lost my job—"through no fault of my own". On one such occasion I was so incensed and angry that I could not even pass the premises in a car without literally wanting to vomit. A couple of months later, however, not only had we won a civil claim for constructive dismissal and garnered a handy compensation payment, but I was offered a new, better-paid job in the accountancy firm that acted for the company who had sacked me, and around the same time the money for the herbal medicine training course I wanted to do was deposited into my account—that story was related earlier in my preface to this book.

When a new direction presents itself, we must frequently let go of the things that are not meant to be part of that direction. Sometimes the letting go needs to happen first, before the new event presents itself. It's a bit like the detox principle of cleansing before rebuilding, discussed in Chapter 1.

It is glib to counsel people to remain calm in adversity (like the popular motto, "Keep Calm and Carry On"). It is intuitive to shout, rage, curse and rant. It's even understandable to some extent to want to go out and punch the people responsible (I hasten to add I am talking about *feelings* here—I am not inciting violence!). It's therapeutic, to some extent, to indulge feelings that offer us a semblance of power in a situation in which power has been taken away from us. However, it can also become a default setting to expect the worst: in the words of the Wet Wet Wet song, "Why does it always rain on me?" (the band name itself seems to identify the problem!)

Pessimism, negative self-dialogue and poor self-regard, expecting the worst, being "down on oneself", potentially have more far-reaching effects than we commonly realise, and in the weird and wonderful world of psychoneuroimmunology are regarded as part of the aetiology of very physical complaints. Cardiovascular disease, autoimmune inflammatory conditions, gastrointestinal dysfunction, and even cancer, have all been associated with disturbed patterns of self-dialogue, and if you are unfortunate enough to suffer from one of these complaints you will be very familiar with the phenomenon of stress-related aggravation of your condition.

Perturbations of mind, emotions and spirit are therefore to be taken entirely seriously as part of the pathophysiology of disease—indeed, if you break the word down to its component parts, dis–ease, you get the picture. The concept of "stress-related" illness is commonplace now, but even with this understanding, few realise how deep this goes. It would not be an exaggeration to say that there is no physical condition that you can have that does not have an emotional or psychic component. More than that, in energetic systems of health theory, these effects are arguably primary and causative, rather than being mere additional symptoms owing to the effects of being ill.

Mind and body are a continuum. In fact, the concept that we "have" a mind, and, separately, a body, is a perspective limited to our cultural milieu and defined by our uniquely European history and philosophy. In other cultures, especially those whose links to their ancient past have not been severed and discarded, we are first and foremost spirit, or energy, and only secondly "physical".

I have discussed this perspective in depth in my previous book, *The Mind's Eye*, which is about the non-physical applications in Iridology, and consists in a guide to recognising your psychic and emotional constitution as an intimate determinant of your physical patterns of health and disease, and offering a pathway to working with psychological material, not through "therapy", but simply in the understanding that your emotional triggers and complexes are part of a highly individualised pattern that is inherently designed and purposed to lead you to an understanding of yourself.

In this chapter, however, I want to explore some of the practical ways in which we can help ourselves in moments of psychological and emotional distress, from the vast canon of naturopathic modalities and therapeutic practices. We also need to remember that stress is a two-way street: yes shock, trauma and emotional distress can affect the body, but you will also find that looking after the body and creating relaxation and a sense of well-being will ease the mind in return. More than that, diligent effort spent increasing your level of vitality and resilience by following the practical advice contained in this book will pay untold dividends if, and when, it comes to "the worst". Your stamina, resistance, energy, your ability to self-regulate and assume command and response-ability in whatever scenario you find yourself will have undergone a significant upgrade.

Plant medicine

If we regard plants as alternatives to drugs, we miss the point and we do not give ourselves the opportunity to experience their ability to communicate with our distress at the deepest levels. It is not unusual for people in distress to resort to pharmaceuticals—sedatives, sleeping pills, "antidepressants" and so forth. Your GP will usually be more than happy to assist by means of the prescription pad. Some may find themselves self-medicating with alcohol and tobacco (how many times in the past did I take up smoking again after a catastrophic relationship fail?), as well as so-called "recreational" street drugs.

What I am suggesting in reaching out to the plant world is not the same-old, same-old need for avoidance and unconsciousness, but something far deeper and more satisfying—more *healing*, in fact. The herb St John's wort (*Hypericum perforatum*) gained a reputation as an "antidepressant" after an article was published in the *Lancet* (the journal of the British Medical Association) comparing it favourably with Prozac as a treatment for mild to moderate depression. The shelves of health food stores around the country were emptied of St John's wort products almost overnight, not only by people self-medicating, but by GPs recommending patients to go and buy the herb rather than take prescription pharmaceuticals.

In traditional medicine, St John's wort is a vulnerary, which means it heals wounds. We might say it is a *trauma healer*, and that it may heal the trauma of the mind and emotions, as well as those of the body. It is also hepatic (acts on the liver to assist detoxification), hypnotic (induces sleep) and nervine (relaxes and strengthens the nerves). I challenge Prozac to do all that!

In Chinese medicine terms it would probably be called a *Shen* tonic—the word Shen can perhaps be most simply translated as "spirit", although it is somewhat more complex than that. Shen tonics are herbs that have the very special property of calming the mind and helping to ease the tribulations of life. They do so by nourishing the heart (the seat of the "Shen" in the Chinese system)—not just the physical heart but the emotional heart too. In Western herbal medicine they might be described as *thymoleptics*—mood-enhancers. Here are some more plants that have those properties:

- Lemon balm (*Melissa officinalis*)—grows prolifically pretty much everywhere, in fact if you have it in your garden you need to use it as it will take over quite readily if not cut back. The easiest way to use it is as a very beautiful aromatic tea—simply rub a handful of leaves between your hands, drop the leaves into a mug, and pour hot water over them. **NB: do not use this herb if you have an underactive thyroid.**
- Rose (*Rosa damascena*)—the Damask rose, the mother of all ornamental roses wherever they are found, is one of the best heart tonics in the plant kingdom. Dubbed by one class of my students many years ago as a "hug in a bottle" (the name has stuck, and spread), it can act very quickly to settle an inflamed mind and ease a troubled breast. Take as a tincture—10 to 15 drops are usually enough, but you can repeat this as often as you need to. Rose is also a great hepatic (liver herb), having a *pacifying* action on that organ, and we have already made the connection between the liver and stress.
- Siberian ginseng (*Eleutherococcus senticosus*)—I almost hesitated to put this herb into the list as there are sustainability issues affecting it at the current era. However, it has been a personal ally of mine for many years, and I still use it to assist at moments of exhaustion, low mood, and the need for stamina and resistance in overcoming adversity. It is classified as an adaptogen, which means it helps us to deal with stress. Closely associated with this herb is Rhodiola, also a Siberian plant, that once got itself a reputation as the "alternative St John's wort". Adaptogens are in the front line of plants chosen for their ability to assist in times of hardship, physical or mental, and many of them are also immune strengtheners, adrenal tonics, nootropics (they support brain function), reproductive tonics and aphrodisiacs!
- Codonopsis (*Codonopsis pilosula*)—another adaptogen, sometimes unkindly referred to as "poor man's ginseng" because it is cheaper and easier to access, and does most of the things ginseng does ... except I think of this plant as a wonder in itself. Its pinyin name is

Dang Shen, which translates roughly as "state of the spirit". I have found that the benefits of using this plant in those stressed to the point of crisis are unparalleled.
- Rosemary (*Rosmarinus officinalis*)—another plant that is easy to cultivate, and one that has so many uses—digestive aid, cardiovascular stimulant, thyroid tonic, cerebral circulatory stimulant and brain tonic. I even think this herb might be a candidate for a Western adaptogen (noting that most herbs in this category tend to be exotic, usually Asian plants in current herbal literature). Its main benefit in times of stress is its ability to promote clarity of thought, while at the same time relaxing the thinker!

Once again, there are so many plants that didn't make it into this list—many of you will have your favourites. Look also at the list of plants mentioned in the section on sleep (Chapter 5). If you haven't yet experienced the benefits of plant medicines to help in these situations then select a couple to get to know. You'll be glad if you do ever get the opportunity to put them to the test.

The Bach Flower Repertory

Edward Bach (1886–1936) was a medical doctor, pathologist and bacteriologist who spent the early years of his career working on vaccines and performing early research on the microbiota of the gut and its connection with chronic disease. In this latter endeavour he was clearly ahead of his time, however he also aspired towards a more holistic treatment paradigm than that offered by standard medicine, and in the latter years of his life he developed his Repertory of the Bach Flower Remedies, partly based on homeopathic principles. These plants were carefully selected for their ability to address the non-physical, emotional and spiritual aspects of healing.

Bach regarded his repertory as fully complete with its 38 remedies, but since then other essences have also made an appearance on the market, most notably the Australian Bush Flower Remedies. The idea behind "plant essences" is firmly rooted in the assumption that physical disease is predicated upon energetic and vibrational disharmony that is also expressed through emotional distress. In my own earliest encounter with natural healing, I was also treated with Bach Flower essences, and I can attest to the beautiful subtlety of feelings that they evoked, quite unlike anything else I had experienced.

The practice starts with identifying key emotional descriptors, such as "fear of unknown origin", or "carrying the weight of the world on your shoulders", and then selects the remedy that resonates with that vibration and is able to neutralise it and insert a positive emotion in its place.

You can buy the full repertory, with explanatory text and instructions for use, from the Bach Centre;[1] however, it may be better to experience them first through consulting with a Bach Flower practitioner. In my day it was also common to give the remedy without telling the patient what was in it. That way any preconceived expectations were ruled out, and the patient could respond to the experience from the pure consciousness of its effects. I am not certain that this is still the preferred practice, but personally if I give Bach remedies, which I do from time to time, this is how I will generally do so—with the consent of my patient of course.

In the context of addressing sudden traumatic distress the Bach system offers the famous Rescue Remedy. I strongly recommend that you keep this remedy handy in your home medicine chest at all times.

Physical movement

We have dealt with movement as a means of enhancing and preserving health in general terms. Here I am keen to introduce it as a means of managing stressful episodes in life and helping individuals to navigate their own trauma.

Afflictions of the mind and emotions are all too often dealt with using a very cerebral approach, often embodied in various systems of "psychotherapy". Although some of these do indeed start to reach into bodily experience (see below section on bodywork), they can also be circular and unproductive, depending upon intellectual knowledge that is not so well-grounded in physical experience.

The importance of the physical is that very often this is the level on which we do most of our processing. The originator of German New Medicine, Ryke Geerd Hamer,[2] proposed that all physical diseases have the function of processing difficult psychological and emotional material—trauma—that the individual cannot easily withstand, mentally. He called diseases "special biological processes of nature", and he stated very strongly that surgical removal and chemical poisoning risks interrupting their healing purpose.

Getting "into the physical" when badly affected emotionally has the advantage of shifting awareness away from relentless circular rumination and giving the mind another focus. Physiologically it also changes both endocrine and neurological chemistry, opening up the creative, problem-solving centres of the brain such as the hippocampus, and presenting new perspectives to the struggling mind.

Nowhere is this more evident—and vital—than in the case of serious psychiatric illness: severe depression, personality disorders, bipolar disease and schizophrenia are all conditions that can be helped by grounding in tough physical activity, which has the effect of pulling the focus of consciousness back into the body and away from the perceived locus of trauma and distress—the mind. Going for a long walk, or even a run, or engaging in vigorous exercise of any denomination, can be a highly effective strategy for dealing with any case of emotional upheaval and psychological distress. It can also help with sleep, which can be severely disrupted at times of extreme stress.

Self-described "urban shaman" Gabrielle Roth's "5-Rhythms" dance practice takes the body through a wave-like cycle of kinaesthetic experience taking in slow, gentle and flowing movements, to staccato, spiky posturing, vigorous and chaotic catharsis, and back again through lyrical and poetic expressions to stillness. The whole sequence is done to an appropriate choice of musical compositions, some specifically designed for this work, and can take two hours to complete the cycle. It is a complete practice and form—movement medicine—which nonetheless gives full range for individual interpretation of the various "rhythms" featured.

Twelve years after Roth's death, as I write, 5-Rhythms groups can be found up and down the country in the UK run by people who trained with Gabrielle. I myself, with my partner, attended some of her London workshops, one of which was a week-long marathon. One of the advantages of her style and practice is that there is no baseline of agility or accomplishment needed to take part. Experienced practitioners dance alongside complete beginners, disabled people beside able bodies. All that is necessary is the willingness to explore yourself through movement, using the prescribed rhythms.

Bodywork

Bodywork is an umbrella term for a variety of practices that exert an effect upon the physical body, usually by means of manual contact. It can include:

Massage
Aromatherapy
Physiotherapy
Osteopathy
Chiropractic
Craniosacral therapy
Bowen technique
Bioenergetics
Feldenkrais method
Heller work
Alexander technique
Deep tissue massage
Rolfing
Fascial release
Polarity Therapy
Acupuncture
Acupressure
Shiatsu
Amatso
Reflexology
Thought Field Therapy
Emotional Freedom Technique

… and doubtless many more. Some of these methods are explicitly psychodynamic in focus, aiming to bring about awareness of emotional content by unlocking the bodily repositories of those energies: the popular mantra is, "The issues are in the tissues", and the theory is that by bringing them into awareness and releasing them physically, they can also be released emotionally.

An advantage of bodywork is, once again, the focus is not the emotion or the distress but the bodily experience—whether "negative" (pain, stiffness, tension) or "positive" (relaxation, warmth, tingling). The more the patient can let go into the experience the better, and that factor itself may be responsible for a good proportion of the benefit derived from such therapies. To have the opportunity to surrender to therapeutic touch in a situation of trust and relaxation is one of the deepest benefits that humans can offer to each other, and is also known to stimulate the all-important pro-social hormone, oxytocin, which plays significant roles in human behaviour including social bonding and connection, romantic love, reproduction and of course childbirth. It is one of the most powerful ways I know to help people, and to be helped by them.

Purpose, and a path with heart

My teacher, the Herb Doc, once advised us, if you ever find yourself waking up not looking forward to your day, you should probably think about stopping what you are doing and make some different plans. Being fully signed up to your path in life can get you through a multitude of hardships—probably you will have had to traverse difficulties in pursuit of your path in the first place. Having a purpose and a passion in life is both challenging and rewarding. The challenge comes from the realisation that anything worthwhile probably needs to be pursued vigorously and persistently; the reward from the knowledge that this is your path, and the certainty that this gives you in respect of the meaning of your life. But the reward is not something you need to wait for: it comes *with* the certainty, in tandem with the work that you perform in its pursuit.

Personally, I believe that if you are on this planet, you are here for a reason. No one else can tell you what that reason is, but if you don't *know* the reason, then life can seem aimless and full of anxiety and uncertainty. For three consecutive years now, I have worked in the Healing Field at the famous Glastonbury Festival of the Arts in Somerset, UK, giving Iridology sittings for festival goers. I mainly use the "Quantum Iris Analysis" method described in my book *The Mind's Eye*, which gives access to these dimensions of a person's life. The hypothesis is, if you are here for something specific, then you might very well be equipped with the qualities, attributes and aptitudes that you need for the purpose, as nothing is random or accidental in this universe. All we then need to do is read those criteria in the irides (plural of iris) and use that for the basis of a discussion about what, potentially, you might do with them.

Almost all the people I worked with in that situation were in a state of suspension in terms of their life direction: considering changing jobs (in one case having given up her job before making any alternative plan), listlessly jumping from one job to another, not believing in their ability to make their dreams come true. All of them, however, once we started to get down to the serious discussion, knew what they wanted to do, and what their purpose was.

It was not hard to discover. I just asked them questions such as, what did they always know they wanted to do when they were younger? In which direction do their thoughts turn in moments of reverie and contemplation? And if money and opportunity were no object, what would they most like to spend their time doing? There was no doubt and no confusion—just a curious disconnect between the object of their desire, and the thought that maybe that was something they ought to be pursuing.

If you are disconnected from your heart's desire you will not be happy, and if you are not happy, the chances are you will not be truly healthy. It doesn't even have to be your job, in terms of livelihood, but it should feature prominently in your life. Plenty of people make a perfectly acceptable bargain between the exigencies of paying the bills, and those of fulfilling a creative or vocational passion. Sometimes indeed that works out better: the root of the word "amateur", for example, is the Latin *Amo*—I love. Amateurs do what they do out of pure love and passion, and are by no means always the unaccomplished, second-rate performers that the word has come to signify.

I have known "famous", successful people, especially in the music business (since that has also been an aspiration of mine) who felt trapped, unfulfilled and unable to pursue their true creative direction precisely *because* they were famous and successful and were too busy living up to the expectations that their success had generated to connect with their deeper instincts. Some of them have become my students and pursued an altogether different direction.

I am completely OK with the fact that I never attained rock and roll stardom. The dream was never to be a "star" anyway. The dream was to write and play music, and I do. I even earn money from it. I am an "amateur" in the best sense of the word, but I tell people that I am a professional, because I am, in all meaningful senses of *that* word. (You can have more than one profession—that's another little secret they won't tell you.)

To follow a path with heart is a declaration that it doesn't matter what that path is, as long as *your* heart is in it. That's all that matters. And the reason why it matters is that if you do not fulfil your purpose on this earth, there's no one coming to rescue you or make amends. Remember those three "pillars" of natural healing from Chapter 1: simplicity, responsibility and change? They can translate to any area of discussion in this book. In the present discussion we might say, the simplicity of knowing what your purpose is; the responsibility to pursue it; and the willingness to make changes in support of it.

Happiness is a big word. I used to distance myself from it. If asked, "Are you happy?" I'd respond, "Who is?" I was a miserable sod, not to put too fine a point on it. Being a wordsmith (pedant), I was also concerned with precise definitions, and I did not really know what it meant. Other words seemed more intuitive—contentment, equanimity, even just "feeling OK". I also held that no emotion was a permanent fixture, so to "be" happy was meaningless as no one could possibly embody that other than temporarily.

All of that was, and is, true. However, as time goes on, I have realised that basically, in ways that I almost never thought possible, I am in fact happy. When I consider what contributes to this, I think it is a basic philosophical orientation. I am not religious, but I think I understand what it is that religion can offer, at its best, and notwithstanding all the judgment, warmongering, prohibition and intolerance: an unshakeable faith that, as St Julian of Norwich puts it in her *Revelations of Divine Love*, "All shall be well, all shall be well, and all manner of thing shall be well."

If I were to prescribe a pathway to this certainty, I would cite my commitment to Natural Healing as the catalyst. Natural Healing assumes that something greater than me is at cause, and in charge, and in my work I see the evidence of that almost daily.

Relationships: Needing the eggs

I have left this topic till last. Relationships are probably going to cause you more grief than anything else in the world. On the other hand, they are also probably going to deliver more joy and fulfilment than anything else. That is probably because they are arguably the single most important reason for being here in the first place. Relationships are the basis of human—or any—social structure, and are forged across many and varied exigencies, from the need for cooperation in the joint projects of survival and creativity, to the bonds that build families and communities, and ensure (ideally) a safe space for procreation, recreation and creativity. There is not enough space in this volume adequately to cover the parameters of "relationship difficulties". There are many commentaries, and many perspectives, theories and methods when it comes to solving them.

The cynical perspective on intimate relationships is well expressed in the joke from the Woody Allen film, *Annie Hall*, about the man who tells his doctor that his brother thinks he's a chicken. The doctor says, "Why don't you turn him in?", to which the brother responds, "I would, but I need the eggs." The Woody Allen character in the film comments, "I guess that's how I feel about relationships. You know they're totally irrational and crazy and absurd, but I guess we keep going through it because we need the eggs." The clever thing about the original joke is that clearly the man is as deluded as his brother. So it often is in relationships, especially when things get contentious: there's no right and wrong in most of these situations, ultimately, simply a tangle that gets tighter the more you tug at the strings.

From a health perspective, if your relationships are giving you grief, they need sorting out. It is often abundantly clear in interviewing patients that their fundamental problem, and the one thing that is preventing them from healing, is a relationship that isn't working. I am not a relationship counsellor (although I have done that job in the past—for a very limited period at a time in my life when I badly needed help in that department myself—which didn't work out too well), and so I offer no advice here, other than this:

When it comes to relationships, of whatever denomination, be fully honest: about your feelings, about your needs, about your wishes. Avoiding this necessity will simply postpone and protract the pain, and potentially create a crisis at some point up ahead in time, when the matter becomes finally and completely intolerable, and can no longer remain hidden.

If you have a good relationship, nurture it. Be attentive, practise tolerance and respect for the other person; be quick to own up and apologise when you make a mistake; and above all, practise seeing the divinity in that person, which is a reflection of your own divinity and worth.

Endnotes

1. https://bachcentre.com.
2. https://learninggnm.com/documents/hamerbio.html.

CHAPTER EIGHT

Cautions, contraindications, and confidence

In this chapter we allow ourselves to question some of the foregoing context. It is important to be able to think on one's feet, and not to get too "hard and fast" about anything where health is concerned. Other factors might be at play, and we might not have all the information we need to hand.

This is about the interface between the Natural Healing perspective and the world of orthodox, or standard health care. How far can Natural Healing take us in our quest to manage our health issues "in house"? I have made a few bold statements about what can be accomplished, and never far beneath the surface of my theory is an incisive critique of standard modern "scientific" medicine. And yet you will also have noticed, I hope, that I refrain from the suggestion that the pure Natural Healing path is for everyone. In fact, I'd even argue that there is no such thing as a "pure" natural healing path in today's world. The three cases discussed below demonstrate my own learning in this respect.

In the end, how far you can go with these methods is for you to decide, but you must be fully realistic—about your own knowledge and skills, about the severity of any particular case, about your own best interests when the dimensions of your situation have all been taken into account and their likely outcomes calculated, and last but not least, about your level of resilience and tenacity when the going gets tough. Far too often I come across well-meaning, but stubborn and sometimes arrogant people, who are dangerously over-confident about their abilities in delivering "natural" solutions: this applies particularly in cases of life-threatening chronic degenerative diseases, such as cancer.

It is not my intention to deal with the subject of cancer in any depth in this book: it is an advanced professional training topic. I absolutely support the possibility of dealing with cancer naturally—if I were ever diagnosed I know which path I would take. I do have a lot of cancer patients—indeed they seek me out for the specialised skills and knowledge that I have. But I have to say that not many of them opt for 100% "natural": most choose an integrated path, and there is some justification in clinical research for this option. From the practitioner point of view there are also issues around legality and the perception and reception of what you may or may not have given your patient to understand. There is a very fine line to tread between being fully positive and empowering, and giving false hope. When we examine the question of health beliefs in Chapter 10 some of the reasons for this will come into perspective.

But I do think it appropriate to place before the reader some examples of situations that may challenge the "natural" perspective, and how they have been handled, to enable you to calibrate your responses and find your own level with this material.

How far are you prepared to go?

This question is not intended to dictate a specific response. Perhaps you believe that the best route forward for you is some kind of integration—Natural Healing, and the best that standard medicine has to offer? That may well work for you—for a time at least. I have seen patients benefit from this approach many times. Part of the reason it works is their sincere belief that it <u>will</u> work, for them: the placebo effect, if you like. The blend of different methods has their full confidence, and that "confidence trick" can be the most important feature in anyone's choice of action. Again, we will tackle the question of health beliefs in the next chapter.

Because the focus of this book is resolutely upon activating the self-healing mechanism within our bodies, I have refrained largely from presenting a fully expanded critique of standard medicine—I have said plenty about it elsewhere, as have many others. While we must consider that methods of disease management that rely upon suppression and the erasing of effects considered undesirable (symptoms) may have hidden dangers, we must also understand that to undermine a patient's confidence in his physician, even if you yourself can clearly see his shortcomings, is likely to be counter-productive, and we need to remember that the vital energy, which in fact does the healing, is always active and can never be discounted in any situation.

It is always a nuanced affair, and each case is deserving of full consideration and a response appropriate to the case. The following cases and accompanying discussions are given in order to provoke some critical thought.

Case 1: Iatrogenic illness: Putting your money where your mouth is

The term "iatrogenic" means, caused by doctors. According to a survey published by the NIH (National Institute of Health) in 2017,[1] medical error accounts for just over a quarter of a million deaths annually in the USA, suggesting, as some were keen to advertise, that it is the third leading cause of death in that country after cardiovascular disease and cancer. Quibbles have taken place over these statistics, and I am not here to confirm or dispute them. They do however suggest that there may be a problem, and in years of practice as a natural healer I have certainly seen evidence of this. It can be subtle and difficult to prove, and doctors at least are fully indemnified against the one clear risk that their profession involves them in: PEOPLE DO DIE. It is simply not possible to save them all. The assigning of blame may seem intuitive if you or a loved one is involved, but it is rarely productive—even if medical fault is proved.

In my own profession I have been involved with cases of complaints being brought against natural health practitioners who have supposedly made errors of judgement. None were upheld as malpractice, and hardly any were firmly established as negligence. My own view, which some might find harsh, is that in matters of health and medicine we each take our chances with the choices we make—the age-old principle of *caveat emptor*: "buyer beware". That of course does not mean that cases should not be appropriately investigated, and channels always exist by which this can be accomplished, in natural medicine as in standard medicine; and we are all required to have a commensurate level of insurance—although I have never in over 30 years of full-time professional practice seen an insurance pay-out in the context of natural medicine.

Our first case concerns a person well-known to me, but not my patient; we will call him Roland. Aged 93, and suffering from severe osteoarthritis of both hips, for which he had had one replacement already and was in the running for another, he had gone for a pre-surgery check-up and was found to have atrial fibrillation. This meant that he was not eligible for surgery, which was a huge disappointment. Following this he awoke one day unable to walk—which he at first thought was due to the deterioration of his hip, but in fact turned out to be a huge pooling of fluid in his lower extremities caused by undiagnosed heart failure. He was quickly brought into hospital where a pleural effusion (fluid on the lung) was also diagnosed.

In the course of investigations, the consultant on his case admitted that the drug regime he had been on (including a calcium-channel blocker for high blood pressure, which inhibits calcium influx to the heart muscle thus diminishing its contractile force) was inappropriate for him, and thus instigated a new regime—Digoxin to address the heart failure (specifically by pumping more calcium into the heart muscle) and furosemide as a diuretic to remove the excess fluid from his lungs and his ankles. His situation stabilised almost immediately, and from being "not expected to leave hospital" and discussing end-of-life care with his wife, he was returned home in a stable condition in just over a week.

Roland was lucky. A lifetime of trust in standard medicine had after all got him to the age of 93, with most of his faculties intact—certainly there was nothing wrong with his cognitive abilities. Mobility was the biggest issue, but a lifetime of suffering with immune-related difficulties—atopic (allergic) conditions such as hay fever and asthma—had also been met with abundant medication.

You might well observe, as do I, that if you can get to the age of 93 using standard medicine as your go-to, that's not a bad recommendation. A lifelong scientist himself, albeit in a completely different sphere of knowledge, Roland believed implicitly in the scientific method. But he knew, and was unhappy, that someone had made a miscalculation that had almost cost him dearly.

Evidence exists that "gold standard" pharmaceutical protocols for managing high blood pressure may be involved in hastening, if not actually causing, congestive heart failure, but doctors have to abide by the standard treatment options allowed to them in the policies and protocols dictated by institutions such as NICE. Once on such a protocol, patients are often told, it's for life. You'll never NOT be on medication again. And that—far too often—is that. If you report feeling unwell on your medication your doctor will search for a suitable analogue—another species or brand of the same medication that hopefully you won't "react" with. But they will not generally change the direction of treatment.

And so you continue, faithfully taking the medicine, until one day, "whoops!"… it turns out that it may have made you more sick than you were before. Small wonder one of the most frequent questions that I hear from the chronically sick when they consult me is, "Is there a way for me to come off these drugs?" And it is my responsible duty to have to explain to them that, if that indeed were possible, it would be a lengthy process, and one which would demand commitment to making far-reaching and meaningful life changes; and that, once the body is used to the drugs, sudden withdrawal may be catastrophic.

It is very rarely the case, as most people seem to believe, that you can simply swap out a herb or a supplement for a drug. Sometimes this can work, but you need to know what you are doing, and it must be carefully monitored; even then there is the long journey to retrace the steps by which you became ill in the first place, to reinstate a natural homeostatic balance.

We are supposed and expected to be on pharmaceutical drugs as we age through life. I call this the "pharmocentric society": pills for ills, and then pills to counteract the ills caused by the pills, and pills to counteract those ills, and so on and on. The highest amount of prescription medicines that I have been asked to assess in a patient, usually dumped unceremoniously in a heap on my desk from a plastic carrier bag, is thirty-one. Thirty-one different pharmaceutical prescriptions for just one patient.

It's all part of the aging process, we are told, and we are grateful that the pharmaceutical companies are there to extend our lives so expertly. Many of the people in this situation, however, are living a kind of half-life, constantly in and out of surgeries and hospitals for one reason or another, collecting another pathology with virtually every visit, held together (barely) by a cocktail of drugs whose side effects and interactions are quite probably incalculable. You can last a long time like this, for sure, but not many people seem to enjoy it, unsurprisingly.

Even in situations like this, however, radical change in a positive direction can be very quickly effective, in the scheme of things, and is always beneficial. American cardiologist Dean Ornish has demonstrated that with a change of diet, and of emotional attitude and approach, even life-threatening cardiac disease can be turned around in less than 12 months, without drugs.[2] His message is simple and empowering: <u>everyone</u>, irrespective of supposedly limiting parameters such as age and genetics, can achieve this level of change in their lives if they commit to it.

Age in particular is a conditioning factor in the minds of many, and assumptions about the psychological flexibility of the "aged" abound in our society. I see this frequently in my younger students, who if asked a question on treating the aged will often roll out platitudes such as, "They are very set in their ways, you know," or "It's unreasonable to expect them to make too many changes." I then ask them, what do you consider old, and they tell me, "Oh anything over 60", or, "Around about 70 years old". I then tell them that I turn 70 next year.

I chose Roland's story because many of his problems are also potentially my problems. I also suffered from atopic conditions for much of the first three decades of my life; at a certain point I also developed high blood pressure; and after a series of accidents left me with multiple musculoskeletal problems, I also developed near-crippling arthritis in one of my hips. Where we differ is in the choices I have made in respect of these issues. At the time of writing I am engaged in the project of healing my hip naturally, and I am making good progress. Someday, if granted sufficient time, I will write the book.

I do not mean to imply that my choices are superior to Roland's. I have yet to demonstrate, after all, that I can make it to 93 years old. Whether I do or do not, however, is not the point. Natural Healing for me is not just a choice of medicine: it is a whole philosophy and a lifelong commitment. As you will have noticed, it extends into many related areas of life—notably spirituality, politics, ecology and sustainability—and it is never something for which I will apologise, even while I fully recognise that it will not be everyone's choice. I genuinely have no judgements about those whose choices are different, but if they come to me for help I will deliver as well as I am able, with the benefit of many decades now of practical experience.

So, when I ask, how far are you prepared to go, I am genuinely interested in your answer. For me, it became an article of faith at a certain point not to visit standard doctors. Not because I judged them poor practitioners or untrustworthy people, or because I had learned over time that, for me, their "solutions" were unsatisfactory; but more positively, because I had proved to my own satisfaction that natural healing methods were both practical and successful.

However, in the interests of balanced reporting, I also had a handful of experiences at the hands of natural medicine practitioners that almost tripped me up. On one occasion a well-respected practitioner visiting from the USA advised me to "take an Advil" for my hip pain (Advil is an American brand of the non-steroidal anti-inflammatory drug ibuprofen). In another incident I paid £300 for an osteopathic assessment of my hip issue, only to be told, "Visit your GP and ask to be put on the list for surgery." Needless to say I declined the advice.

In these cases, the perceived incurability of my condition was the driving force in the advice being given. This has always been a red flag to me—not to mention a red rag! But in the end, I thank these practitioners for incentivising me to intensify my own research, as a result of which I discovered powerful natural pain relief methods, and manipulative techniques that had demonstrated clinically confirmed results in regenerating cartilage (technically, "halting cartilage wear and tear", but by implication, upon close reading, by naturally stimulating cartilage production), among so much more—for another volume. Long story short, six years ago I was reduced to walking with a stick, and even then with difficulty. Four years ago I threw it away for good. Actually I still have it. I keep it in the back lobby in my house, where it acts as a constant reminder of my progress.

Case 2: Emergency medicine—a case apart?

I am often asked by people who have suffered physical trauma—accidents—whether they should visit the hospital, or try to heal themselves "naturally". My first observation is that trauma can be complicated, and it would be important to know the precise extent and parameters of the injury, and we don't always know exactly how things will develop even in the immediate future. Correct expert assessment is of the essence. Even in our most radical natural healing classes with Dr Schulze we were taught that, among the elements of standard medicine that are potentially useful, emergency medicine features most prominently. My advice is generally to let the surgeons do what they do best. We can bring herbs and nutrients to bear once you have had the situation appropriately cleaned up and everything put back in its proper place.

The story is told of the anthropologist Margaret Mead, who when asked by a student what she considered the first evidence of civilisation, replied that in her view it was the archaeological find of a 15,000 year-old broken femur that had healed. She pointed out that in the animal kingdom a broken leg is a sentence of death: you cannot run from danger, you cannot hunt or gather food, you are in effect "meat for your predators":

> A broken femur that has healed is evidence that another person has taken time to stay with the fallen, has bound up the wound, has carried the person to safety and has tended them through recovery. A healed femur indicates that someone has helped a fellow human, rather than abandoning them to save their own life.[3]

Having myself experienced a few significant injuries, I find myself of the opinion that it is best not to take chances with serious physical trauma. This represents something of a sea change for me, as I need also to say that my students' naïve faith in what I might be able to accomplish probably owes itself to a particular story that in the past I have been proud to relate.

It involves Dr Schulze, on one of his deeply anticipated teaching visits to the UK in 1994. My partner was on a two-week training retreat in the North of England, taught by the Doc. I was heading up for the final weekend, proudly driving my newly renovated classic sports car and enjoying the chance to take it on the road for a reasonably substantial run. The weather was treacherous, however, and driving through the Yorkshire Dales on a winding country road, my wheels lost their grip on a bend and the car strayed into the path of an oncoming Range Rover, much bigger than my car, and, as it turned out, pretty much indestructible, for whereas the Range Rover suffered minor damage to the grille, my car was rendered instantly concertina-shaped.

Dazed and confused, I walked out of the wreckage, somehow having the presence of mind to rescue the licence disk from the windscreen, which had popped out fully intact on impact—lucid enough, bizarrely, to realise that the police, who were undoubtedly on their way, would want to see it. When the emergency services arrived on the scene, they approached my vehicle with metal shears expecting to have to cut me out. Finding no one in the driver's seat—"Where's the driver of this vehicle?"—they were startled when I tapped them on the shoulder and said, "Here I am." "You got out ... of THIS?" they exclaimed incredulously. I shrugged. I felt fine ... I was of course actually the walking wounded fuelled on sheer adrenalin, perfectly convinced that I could continue my journey to see Dr Schulze, whose reputation from the many stories he told of dealing with his own traumatic injuries reassured me that he would undoubtedly be able to advise on the treatment of any minor ill effects accruing from this mishap.

I refused the ambulance ride into hospital (I had to sign a disclaimer), convinced that I was basically OK and that Dr Schulze would be the man to help me repair my injuries naturally, so instead I took a ride in a police car to the conference centre where the seminar was taking place. I walked in and explained that I had just been in an accident, and needed to see Dr Schulze. I was set down in the hotel lounge with the traditional cup of hot, sweet tea, and I relaxed.

It was at that point that I knew I was in bigger trouble than I had suspected. Lifting my hand from where it was resting on my knee, I noticed that it was dripping with blood, and that the blood was not coming from my hand, but seeping through my trousers from my knee. The shock hit me like a wave and I had to be carried to my bedroom and laid out on the bed while my clothing was carefully removed. The laceration in my knee was about 3 centimetres across, a deep circular gouge, right down to the patella—in fact a chunk of flesh was entirely missing from the wound (I found it later on the inside of my trousers) and the white of the bone was visibly exposed.

I also had broken bones—feet and ribs, fortunately nothing more—but I was covered from head to foot in grazes, scrapes, cuts and bruises. I was pretty beaten up. There was a deep ache in my femur on the same side as the knee injury, and I realised that my leg had been forced into the crumpling dashboard causing the injury, but thankfully stopping short of splintering my femur—that would have been a whole different situation.

You can read the story from Dr Schulze's point of view in his book, *Cures from the Last Chance Clinic*.[4] He never let on at the time how close he was to sending me to the hospital. He was impressive. He checked me over carefully, including ensuring my blood pressure had not dropped and that I was not in danger of suffering shock owing to undiagnosed internal bleeding. With a dozen students of herbal medicine gathered around my bedside as I lay stretched out naked on the bed he examined every inch of me to ascertain that there was nothing of greater concern than the obvious injuries (the seminar on herbal cardiovascular protocols having now been converted to a naturopathic trauma-care class).

This is how he identified the broken bones (feet and ribs do not require setting or plastering so I was OK). My surface wounds were cleansed. With the help of two male students of sufficient size and strength I was lowered into a warm bath containing some powdered cayenne pepper, to stanch any continuing superficial blood loss.

Back on the bed, the knee was dressed with a poultice of herbal powders to provide antiseptic, haemostatic and vulnerary support and covered with a light bandage; and I was given what must have been the first ever UK serving of Dr Schulze's fully organic vitamin and mineral superfood blend, which he had literally just developed and brought with him from the USA. I was given a couple of tubs to take away.

The next morning blood pressure was taken again, and finding me stable and satisfactory, the Herb Doc proceeded to look at the knee laceration, removing the dressing and the poultice. To the astonishment of the assembled students around my bed, the bone of the patella was no longer visible: the flesh had begun to heal, at a super-fast rate. There were two nurses in the group who testified that they had never seen such results, and that a case like this in standard medical terms would arguably need a skin graft.

A fresh poultice was applied together with a small bottle of very potent antiseptic herbal extracts. I was instructed to leave the poultice on until it fell off naturally, but to monitor the edges of the wound, which might suppurate a little, in which case they were to be treated by direct topical application of the antiseptic tincture around the edges of the poultice.

My brother-in-law, Bill, very kindly arrived to transport Anji and myself back home. I was relieved when I saw that his car was a Range Rover.

The other key instruction was at all costs to keep the leg straight until the healing was complete—no splint had been applied as we wanted to keep the wound as lightly dressed as possible. This I did by sheer effort of will for three and a half weeks (a bed was made up for me in the living room so I did not have to negotiate stairs), at which point the poultice duly fell off, leaving a patch of perfectly healed, bright pink flesh. To this day there remains only the faintest of scars to remind me (I frequently forget) which leg was involved (it was the right). I diligently took a twice-daily dose of the Superfood blend to ensure an abundant supply of vital nutrients. Four weeks after the accident I was driving a car again—two weeks in advance of the standard medical advice.

Fast forward fifteen years to my next accident, which was a partial rupture of my right Achilles tendon. Once again I determined that I would see to this naturally, without recourse to medical expertise. The healing again progressed faster than normal, and although I was reckless enough to over-challenge the injury site on a couple of occasions—basically by refusing to stop and rest, resulting in two further abruptions—the results drew an impressed response from the osteomyologist whose help I sought in rehabilitation. He was known for treating professional footballers and had seen similar injuries many times. He told me that it was actually a complex injury involving not only the Achilles, but the soleus muscle (ripped in half) and abruptions of the ligament insertion points around the heel. I had, however succeeded in reestablishing seven-eighths of the original thickness of the Achilles, and had healed most of the other injuries.

Seven-eighths might sound great, but in fact it makes a significant difference to your gait forever afterwards, and has a distinct disadvantage in throwing the burden of compensation over onto the opposite leg. Thus, when consulting osteopaths since that time on the matter of the wear and tear in my left hip, all have confirmed that in their opinion these earlier injuries might have played a significant part in the aetiology of the arthritic condition that later established itself in that joint.

To some extent I buy this, while also having to add the genetic component: both my parents, one of my grandparents and at least two of my siblings also presented with advanced osteoarthritis of the hip. Also to be considered is that even had I gone to the orthopaedic surgeons, the same outcome might have applied. But although the jury is out on the precise causation, and "What if?" is a big, unanswerable question, I know from how things feel in my undercarriage that the damage was not 100% mended. There's been a lot of osteopathy and hatha yoga since that time to maintain the geometry in something resembling optimal alignment—especially since, 2 years later, I also broke my left ankle.

One other small piece of personal history that has been constitutional in my own development: while in my "gap year", preparatory to going to university, I took a job in what was at the time Redhill General Hospital as an Operating Department Assistant (ODA). Back in those days (1973) it was a "casual" job (believe it or not): now it is a skilled profession with appropriate training and qualification.

My job was to maintain the operating theatres (two of them in that hospital at the time), and all their equipment, including the anaesthetic machines, along with the relevant pharmaceuticals. In fact during surgeries my specific role was to support the anaesthetist. It was a highly responsible job, and one which I loved so much that I went and did it again several times during university holidays—and was welcomed back, which I take as a measure that my employers liked me and were very happy with my services.

The specialisms of the hospital were General Medicine (mainly gastrointestinal), Orthopaedics (bones and ligaments), and Obstetrics and Gynaecology (childbirth and women's complaints). But the hospital was also the main accident and emergency (then "Casualty") unit for the surrounding area, and especially on the graveyard shifts, of which I took my fair share, we would be mobilised at the drop of a hat for road traffic accidents (many, of all levels of severity), terrorist attacks (anyone remember the Caterham pub bombing of 1975?), and even aviation-related emergencies (Gatwick airport was in the catchment area).

Consequently I have seen plenty of gruesome injuries, and been personally involved as a member of the team responsible for helping the victims. I have witnessed first-hand the skills of surgeons specialised in this type of work, and I have nothing but respect and admiration for them. In their own way they do perform miracles of healing, and we would be ill-advised to discount their services to our community.

The combined point of these stories is, Natural Healing can accomplish near-miracles, even in the case of traumatic injury, but you need to know what you are doing, or be in the care of someone else who knows. Expert professional advice is essential, and in the end, as the Herb Doc himself said, emergency medicine is the one branch of standard medicine that we can be truly thankful for. We are talking here of significant, potentially life-changing injuries. It's fine to use these methods and principles for the ordinary everyday scrapes and cuts—but again, ensure your assessment of the damage is accurate, and if there is any doubt, seek expert help.

Similar advice applies to cases of sudden health emergencies, such as cardiac arrest or a severe asthma attack. There are stories—some entirely true—circulating about resuscitating people with tincture of cayenne pepper (Dr Christopher reports using several cups of hot cayenne tea until the person comes round). The problems with this in the current era are perhaps too obvious to state, but legality is one. There is only one treatment to be administered by a non-authorised medical person in the case of cardiac arrest: CPR. If after the fact you are discovered to have used a non-standard remedy, you may well be prosecuted.

In most cases in our world today emergency help is not far away, and defibrillators are often found in public spaces and work places. But there is one other glaring reason for NOT using "natural" remedies in such instances: you have NO IDEA what other medication that person may be on, and the risk of triggering an adverse interaction is simply not worth it. Go and get yourself a basic training in emergency first aid, and keep your knowledge updated—every three years is the usual requirement. Once the emergency has been taken care of, the role for Natural Healing in improving long-term outcomes can be discussed and negotiated.

Case 3: A new arrival

Our final case involves obstetrics—childbirth. There are few medical events that carry such a charge, a potential for either rejoicing or regret. The reason that childbirth is routinely medicalised in our age is more than simply that "they" want to control us from cradle to grave. It is borne of a long and traumatic human history of danger and risk associated with childbirth. In Victorian Britain for example, infant mortality in childbirth stood anywhere between 20 and 50 percent—presumably dependent upon social conditions, wealth and other health-determining factors. That's just infant deaths: add maternal deaths and this is a staggering attrition compared with today's figures of 0.5–1% in the developed world.

Despite today's low risk, midwives that I have spoken to have confirmed that insurance companies are reluctant to cover independent midwives specialising in 'natural' and home birthing. The argument is that the low mortality rate is precisely BECAUSE we have medicalised the process of childbirth.

Nonetheless, many natural healing aficionados approaching childbirth, usually with a head charge of idealism, will dogmatically insist on "natural" at all costs. If they know what they are doing, fair enough, but otherwise we should always have an eye on safety and the fact that there is another, unborn, human being at stake, to whom, in the fulness of time, we may have to answer. Natural childbirth is certainly possible, and despite the insurance difficulties mentioned above, there are practitioners who specialise in it, some of them within the NHS. My advice is to seek one out and engage her for the purpose. Such practitioners will be fully trained in what a potential emergency looks like, and ready to transfer to hospital in good time to prevent a catastrophe.

Nevertheless (as you might expect if you are reading our characters rightly through the pages of this book), my partner and I made something of a nuisance of ourselves at the birth of our first child, and caused significant anxiety in those detailed to our case. I spoke briefly about this in my preface, but the birthing took place on a mattress on the floor of our bedroom in a communal house, in the height of a very hot summer where flies and pestilence were never far away. The pregnancy itself had been "textbook", with no complications; nevertheless, the evening before the birthing the lead midwife was so concerned that before she left she had spread newspaper sheets all around the bed.

We had looked at each other with mock horror, wondering what on earth this was supposed to achieve, and as soon as she had gone, we bundled them all up in a ball and discarded them. The night passed peacefully enough, and we were awoken at about 7am with the first proper contractions, and called the obstetric team back in. Our midwife brought two other practitioners with her, one older midwife who remembered home births well from her far earlier experience, and one student midwife, for whom a home birth was such a rare occurrence it was not to be missed. Our son was born at 10.05am with no complications.

Twelve years later we again found ourselves in a birthing situation. Emboldened by previous experience we again specified a "natural" birthing plan. This time the medical team was far more accommodating, and we did not experience a great deal of resistance. Again, the pregnancy was uneventful (medically speaking), and we arrived near the end of the final trimester in state of joyful anticipation.

However, complications arose, firstly around the fact that he went over the due date and, although the waters had broken, there was no sign of contractions. At a certain point the midwife became concerned about the foetal heart-rate and strongly advised a visit to the obstetrics unit at Addenbrookes Hospital. We conceded, and were duly transferred, all the while expecting that they would discharge us within a couple of hours so that the actual birth could take place at home. This they strongly counselled against, nonetheless we eventually did persuade them to release us into our midwife's care.

Shortly after that contractions established themselves, but they were not as enthusiastic as the midwife would have liked, and so the threat of a second transferral was ever-present. It was explain to us that we had 48 hours after the breaking of the waters before transferral would be mandatory. In fact we knew this, as we had covered pregnancy and childbirth in depth in our own training, and even in natural midwifery terms the 48 hours limit was considered absolute. We also knew a full range of herbal and natural techniques for kick-starting contractions, and we deployed them all.

At 47 hours, contractions began in earnest. The midwife judged that she just had time to go home, change and eat, and things would be well underway by the time she got back in just over an hour. Less than a minute after she was gone I heard an urgent shout from our 12-year old. He had been following his mother up the stairs, and had seen that she was gushing with blood. I called the midwife but she was driving and could not answer. I called 999, and an ambulance was duly dispatched.

As we waited, I did the only thing I knew how to do, which was to administer several millilitres of tincture of cayenne pepper, orally, in successive doses by means of a pipette. Cayenne is a superb haemostatic and circulatory equaliser, administered either topically or internally, and it did the trick: the bleeding subsided. The ambulance came, and mother and baby-in-waiting were blue-lighted to the birthing unit. I took pursuit in the car with our son, closely followed by our midwife.

After that the birthing went smoothly. The medical team was sensitive to our disappointment and gave us the best experience we could have hoped for under the circumstances, in a darkened private room, and an atmosphere of calm and reassurance. They were also fully compliant with our stated preferences for minimal pain relief (nitrous oxide and oxygen on standby if needed—it wasn't), delay to the oxytocin injection (to close down the uterus and prevent further blood loss) until after the cutting of the umbilical cord, and baby delivered into my arms, and then to mother's breast.

The birth of a child, under no matter what circumstances, is always a joyous occasion. In my previous experience as an ODA (related above) I was frequently in attendance at Caesarian sections. It was the one surgical procedure that everyone loved to be around, even if necessitated by emergency issues. Our disappointment at the last-minute scuppering of our plans quickly gave way to relief, gratitude and euphoria. But there was more to come. In my heart of hearts I was still asking, "Why? What did we do wrong? Why was this even necessary?" I soon found out.

At a certain point, when mother and baby were settled and sleeping, I was dispatched by the medical team to take our older son home to bed, and to collect all those essentials that we had prepared but had no time to gather before the sudden transferral to hospital. Upon entering our home I was confronted with a scene of devastation. The birthing mattress that we had set up in our living room was covered in debris—masonry, plaster and timber. The ceiling had collapsed. Had we gone ahead with our fiercely desired home birth, we would all have been underneath it when it happened.

If you are spooked reading this, imagine how we felt. Suffice it to say that on the physical plane we sometimes do not have all the information we need when making choices that we think are in our best interests. We need to be prepared to be overturned by fate. In the end, someone had our backs—unseen spirits and angels in the world beyond? The child himself perhaps not fully in the physical but aware of the conditions into which he was about to arrive? This event challenged the rational world view in so many ways. Even today I continue to marvel. But the very clear message is, remain flexible and keep your wits about you. No precept or ideal is worth risking life for.

* * *

There is just one other thing, however, that I want to say in defence of maintaining the knowledge of natural emergency measures. We live in a world where we have become almost terminally dependent on the infrastructure of civilisation—state healthcare and the emergency services, but also including transport, water supplies, basic hygiene and insurance. Were things ever to collapse (there are zones in the world today where this has happened, and is happening as we speak) and these conveniences be no longer available, those who have kept this knowledge alive might find themselves in high demand indeed.

Endnotes

1. https://pubmed.ncbi.nlm.nih.gov/28186008/.
2. Ornish Lifestyle Medicine (2023). *Empowering You*. Available at: https://learninggnm.com/documents/hamerbio.html.
3. Yancey, P. (1987). *Fearfully and Wonderfully Made* (Grand Rapids: Zondervan).
4. Schulze, R. (1995). *Cures from the Last-Chance Clinic: An Introduction to the Methods of an Herbal Master* (Charlottesville: The University of Natural Healing).

CHAPTER NINE

The spectrum of wellness

What has been presented in the foregoing pages is my own take on the knowledge that I have gathered both in my original training and the arguably more extensive training bestowed upon me in more than 40 years of committed practice and personal experience. I hope that the practical advice has been amplified by the commentary, as they do ideally go hand in hand. I have learned through years of working with people that "simple" instructions may yet be misunderstood, or require further clarification, and it is often the benefit of repeated requests for clarity that you are offered here in this book, in addition to the "raw material".

I have hinted a few times that I am not here to tell you what to do, but rather to help you to think through the various issues and come to a conclusion that is right for you. I have introduced a few tools for doing this and tried to guide your thoughts in terms of this little word, NATURAL, and what it means. Further, I have offered the opinion (and it is just my opinion) that you hold the ultimate responsibility for your health, and that to give it away without reserve makes no sense in today's world—if it ever did.

A bit more politics...

I am fond of quoting French philosopher and historian Michel Foucault on this issue. In his book *The Birth of the Clinic* he observes, "Before it became a corpus of knowledge, the clinic was a universal relationship of mankind with itself ... the decline began when writing and secrecy were introduced, that is, the concentration of this knowledge in a privileged group."[1] We are taught to trust doctors. And why not? We assume that human beings want the best for each other and that those whose calling is to help will be of pure intention. I am not saying that medical doctors do not have the very best of intentions—I know many, and I have personally educated many in the ways of Natural Healing. They are on the whole good people who are committed to making a difference.

However, in key respects they have been misled. Medicine is in the grip of a monolithic corporate agenda that may eventually afford it unprecedented power over every human being on the planet, if the current trajectory is allowed to proceed unchallenged. The events of the last four to five years, as I write, have revealed the extent of this agenda of control, at least to those who are paying attention. The agenda, however, is still being developed by stealth. The World Health Organization is on the brink of persuading an overwhelming majority of global states to sign up to its "Pandemic Preparedness Treaty", and although the UK government website distances itself from claims that this would mean handing sovereignty and human rights over to a centralised policy-making body,[2] the writing is most definitely on the wall when it comes to medical freedom, as indeed it is for financial freedom—and the terrifying thing about that is that they will very likely go hand in hand in the future—unless we do something about it.

In his book *The Care Economy*,[3] Tim Jackson handles the gargantuan and multi-level project of analysing exactly why, in the contemporary era, considerations of health and care have come to be secondary to—indeed are the antithesis of—cultural and political homage to the holy grail of economic growth (capitalism) which prioritises wealth over health (and then generally only for the few). Traversing a terrain redolent with stories and examples ranging from the myths of antiquity, the histories of science and medicine, the recent shift in the landscape of health thanks to Covid-19, and gender politics, Jackson highlights the need for, and the possibility of, systemic economic change as a solution to the near-catastrophic failure of "health care" in our time.

Set alongside that, freedom of choice in health care, which is the fundamental freedom to be the sole and sovereign authority in respect of what is done to, or introduced into our bodies, is the highest value that I can support; but it has to be a personal choice, and inevitably there will be many different responses. In the end I am here to persuade, not to dissuade, which is to say that it is an article of faith that I will never override anyone's choice, no matter that their choice would never be my choice. My contention is that it is the informed choices of individuals *en masse* that will be the effectors of social change. They will never give it to us: we have to take it. And that means making new and different choices in our everyday lives—or, as the saying goes, voting with our feet. We cannot wait for the world to change: we are living—or dying—NOW.

That is the difference between the outlook proposed in this book, and one that says, everyone MUST take this medication, everyone MUST be treated the way we dictate. The moment you start behaving like this you become like the very people you might find yourself criticising. Added to that is the fact that standard medicine (as I prefer to call the "modern" variety), which we are supposed to follow without question, does not always rest on the best knowledge we have available. I have discussed this at length in *The Mind's Eye*. Here is a story that demonstrates that.

Although we started our natural healing journey very young, my partner and I were still at a certain era automatically accepting certain practices, for example, routine vaccination. Our first (joint) child received the first round of routine jabs. It was when he was about six years old, and they wrote to us to bring him in for a measles jab, that an alarm went off in our minds. Apparently, since the days of our own childhood—when measles was handled in the community by bringing all the measles sufferers together for a "measles party", which was essentially a way for our parents to cope with the enforced absence from school and the need to look after a bunch of kids who, although spotty, were otherwise clearly in robust health—measles had surreptitiously become a deadly disease that would reportedly kill 1 in every 500 children who contracted it.

At that point I began to research the matter, and having done so I wrote back to the GP to explain that we would not be presenting our son for his measles jab. The letters came and went, and after a while they stopped writing to me, and instead started a campaign of what I can only call terror against my partner. Apparently, they assumed that because she was female and a mother, she would be vulnerable to the fear they sought to instil. We held our ground.

Fast forward six years to the birth of our second son. Noticing after an interval that we had not presented him to the medical authorities to get the standard rites of passage (i.e. his jabs), our GP cycled 5 miles out of the city one evening to come and see us. Our initial surprise and welcome soon turned to suspicion upon hearing her say, "Now, I note you haven't brought him in for his jabs yet. You know you really should consider this. Vaccinations these days are so much *safer* that they were 10 years ago." I said, "Excuse me, but we have a 12-year-old boy in the next room, and he was vaccinated: what are you telling us?"

I am aware that I may be addressing some who not only do not see a problem with vaccination, but who also implicitly believe in it. Here, with no apology, I have to be uncompromisingly true to my own convictions. I used to believe in it—before I looked into the matter in a little more depth. It was always presented as a one-off immune upgrade: introduce your immunity to the pathogen so that it will remember it if it encounters it in the future. What's not to like?

However, at a certain point the narrative began to change: one dose was not enough, you need "boosters". Forgive my scepticism but that to me implies that vaccination does not work as well as we were told? And it takes little account of the innate intelligence of the immune system, which we were originally taught to respect—after all, is not vaccination supposed to work on the basis of priming your immunity to do what it naturally does anyway? Comparing that basic expectation to the rationales deployed in the rolling out of the Pfizer SARS-Cov-19 gene therapy it is obvious that things have indeed "moved on". Our God-given natural immunity, it seems, is now stultified and redundant.

Over the decades more and more diseases started to become "vaxxable" and a belief was slowly engineered into the population that those who did not consent to vaccination constituted a threat to the rest of us. This reached a pitch of fever during the Covid era, in which the unvaccinated became the target of despotic hate (fear) campaigns, some of them conducted by respected intellectual elders who arguably should have known better.[4] It begs the question, if you have been vaccinated, and supposing that this works, how is it possible to be threatened by the unvaccinated, even if they do contract the disease? Surely the whole point of it is, *you* are protected?

Even our GP in the previous story did also say at one point, "Well I guess he will be protected by the fact that everyone else is vaccinated". She was referring to herd immunity. But in 2021, the year that the Covid-19 vaccinations were rolled out, the definition of herd immunity—the theory that an epidemic will naturally burn itself out when enough individuals have achieved natural immunity—was subtly changed. It now came to refer specifically to immunity achieved by vaccination:

> "Herd immunity against COVID-19 should be achieved by protecting people through vaccination, not by exposing them to the pathogen that causes the disease.[5]

In certain states in America a child will typically receive up to 72 inoculations before the age of 2.[6] Far from replicating "natural exposure" to pathogens, this begins to look like a flat-out assault on the developing immune system, not to say an attempt to modify humans in very specific ways, <u>without our fully informed consent</u>, and from a very early age. Consider what else is in these products (let's start with heavy metals such as mercury and aluminium, and "viral components" such as SV40[7]), and from a naturopathic perspective there is credible cause to hypothesise that, far from protecting us, vaccination programs may themselves be contributory factors in the epidemic of non-communicable diseases (including but not limited to chronic and post-viral fatigue syndrome, autoimmune inflammatory diseases, diabetes, Alzheimer's and neurocognitive diseases, cancer, and infertility) that have characterised the late 20th and early 21st centuries—pretty much since vaccines became routine. Coincidence is not the same as causation. But if the possibility exists that, far from creating a healthier population, we are engineering immune dysfunction into humans on a global scale, then we ought to leave no stone unturned in our search for the culprits.

In all probability, of course, we are looking at multifactorial causation, across a range of parameters.

Richard Horton, writing in the Lancet in September of 2020, made the case that Covid-19 should more properly be regarded as a *syndemic* than a pandemic. He points out that rapidly increasing numbers of people in society with NCDs (non-communicable diseases) including diabetes and cardiovascular disease, as well as the consequences of poor health status accruing to below-par living standards, has resulted in widespread susceptibility to poorer outcomes in the face of biological threats such as SARS-Cov-19, and notes:

> *Our societies need hope. The economic crisis that is advancing towards us will not be solved by a drug or a vaccine. Nothing less than national revival*

162   NATURAL HEALING

> *is needed. Approaching COVID-19 as a syndemic will invite a larger vision, one encompassing education, employment, housing, food, and environment.*[8]

I could add here that, were governments and state health care facilities minded to support natural and traditional medicine alongside the standard variety, there is much that could be gained from the methods and insights promoted in this volume. In point of fact, however, as I have noted above in Chapter 1, those of us who were quick to offer advice towards the attainment and maintenance of *natural* immunity and health preservation were actively silenced by the twin interlocking sanctions of deplatforming from social media and personal shaming, discrediting and censure.

Meanwhile, in the orthodox camp itself, all is not quite shipshape. Robert S. Mendelsohn, the author of a brilliant but highly controversial book, *Confessions of a Medical Heretic*,[9] talks about something called the "whoops factor" in medicine. We encountered it earlier in the case of Roland. Medical drugs and procedures are perfectly safe … until they are not. "Ah, we've just found out that it's not quite as safe as we led you to believe. Sorry about that. Never mind, have some (usually inadequate) compensation." The biggest whoops factor in medicine to date has been the thalidomide story. I do not need to repeat the full details here, but a generation of mothers who were persuaded to take this drug to control the symptoms of morning sickness lived to regret their faith in their doctor, and so indeed did many of their progeny.

The biggest, and most often repeated, verdict in relation to the "alternatives"—natural medicine, in effect—is that there is "no evidence" to validate it, and therefore people are instructed by the establishment, through the mainstream media, in the strongest terms, to avoid it. It is perhaps only when you look closely into the question of evidence that you can start to see through this ruse.

Far from being black and white, beyond question and doubt, clinical evidence is itself very much a matter of interpretation—and that's when it is properly conducted. Add into the mix the fairly routine confounding factors, such as medical bias, flaws in the research model, and the cherry-picking of clinical results to "prove" what pharmaceutical companies want you to believe,[10] and you have an edifice of "knowledge", feeding directly into state policy via organisations such as the ironically named "NICE" (National Institute for Clinical Excellence), that is in reality someone's business plan for making a great deal of money at our expense. Small wonder they are trying their best to ridicule, discredit and eliminate the competition.

We live in an age, however, where fear dominates our policies and our practices in relation to medicine and health. Fear of illness, fear of pathogens and viruses, fear of each other, fear of Nature itself. Fear that, without the all-seeing, all-saving grace of modern medicine, we might not survive. Take away people's self-determination and that is all that is left: we are helpless, and therefore we are fearful.

Natural Healing, on the other hand, is not about fear: that's what makes it so dangerous to the status quo; that's why we were deplatformed during the pandemic—not because we were irresponsibly advising people to use "ineffective" and "untested" remedies, but because we were advocating agency and freedom of choice, telling people how they could strengthen their own immunity against the threat. We sought, in fact, to neutralise and offset the fear factor. We may try to sanitise what we do so they think it's OK—the employment of terms such as "complementary" medicine are a means of doing this—but in the orthodox view we are not to be mistaken for *serious* medicine, *proper* medicine, and not to be sanctioned in any way, shape or form when the powers that-be want you to listen up and toe the line.

Sitting in those first Natural Healing classes in the very early days, my mind was lit up with the possibility that Natural Healing was the medicine of the future, as it had been of the past. There was an ethos of "can do" that I got from my teachers, who had variously healed themselves of cancer, auto-immune disease, heart disease and more, using these techniques. The quote from Dr John Christopher, "There's no such thing as an incurable disease" rang loudly in my ears. Later I learned that Christopher himself was quoting Avicenna, the medieval Persian physician, who added, "… *only the want of knowledge*". Was this the knowledge that I felt privileged to acquire, first of all at the tender age of 22, and to develop and practice throughout my working life?

My naivety was short-lived. Since that time I have noticed if anything a doubling down of state-sponsored narratives around medicine, and the development of ever tighter controls over what we are allowed to say about what we do, via institutions such as the Advertising Standards Authority in the UK, who have aggressively and relentlessly hounded practitioners out of business for saying the wrong things on their websites and social media pages. In short, we are gagged—"legally"—when it comes to suggesting that there might be clear medical benefit in anything we do.

In one case, a medical doctor who had retrained with us as a naturopath and a herbalist was arraigned for suggesting that the herb echinacea might help with immune-related problems. She responded by presenting the clinical evidence that it was so. They wrote back telling her that her evidence was inadmissible. The glass ceiling operates even for initiates if they themselves become renegades and go "off narrative". What hope for the rest of us, who no matter how skilled and knowledgeable, no matter how many years spent successfully helping our clients, are still categorised as "lay" when it comes to our professional status?

And yet the sign-up to degree-level training courses in herbal medicine, nutrition, acupuncture, Ayurvedic medicine, homeopathy, osteopathy and naturopathy itself has never been higher. And for all those graduates released into the world as practitioners there appears to be a substantial and growing clientele. Times are changing, but the change is stealthy. It is no good expecting that the governments of the world and the World Health Organization will change the rules in our favour when all the signs are that their intention is to narrow them down even further.

I have spent enough of my personal time at the sharp end of natural medicine politics to know this. I have sat on several professional committees, I have even chaired a few (and still do), and in that capacity I have also sat around negotiating tables opposite civil servants, government ministers, and prominent members of the medical profession, fighting for our future as professional practitioners against restrictive legislation, such as that emanating from the European Union, which in 1994 demanded full "harmonization" of UK law with EU law on the matter of medicines. In many EU states what I do is illegal: it attracts the tag, *practising medicine without a licence*, and it is punishable by imprisonment.

Integrated medicine

Some still believe that the answer is some kind of "integration" with standard medicine. In fact, Integrated Medicine is a growing movement, and I have respect for those who are developing it. It represents one possible direction, and an important choice for those who do not have the requisite knowledge and skills with which to cast off their reliance upon the orthodox medical model, yet who are on a path of discovery with regard to natural or traditional methods. To some extent, as was hopefully evident in the previous chapter, all of us must be prepared to do likewise, especially those of us working as practitioners with the lives of others in our hands.

When patients come into our practice they frequently present with existing diagnoses and ongoing medical treatments. It is our business as professionals to be able to work safely around these treatments, especially pharmaceuticals, where there may be significant interactions and contraindications; and this forms a highly important element in the training of natural medicine professionals in the current era. I'd venture to say that we know more about this dimension of practice than the medics themselves, who get precious little training in what we do, while many natural medicine practitioners on the other hand take biomedicine and clinical pathology up to educational level 6 (BSc degree level) as a routine part of our training.

In countries where "integrated medicine" is well-advanced, however, this has not been found to be free of problems. A study of the experiences of naturopathic practitioners in an Australian integrative health care context found that true integration, together with mutual understanding and respect, is frequently lacking.[11] This failure of integration—poor or reluctant communication, doctors appropriating naturopathic modalities without having understood them properly, medical bias on the part of GPs—impacted negatively on patients themselves and was found to obscure the benefits of the naturopathic treatments that patients were receiving. Standard medicine, in other words, still tends to regard itself as the ultimate authority, and this is something that we need to change.

It is to those who have inherited or developed a similar disposition to mine, however, that the main thrust of this book is directed, and this is a demographic that is rapidly expanding in this era. People will vote with their feet, as standard and conventional protocols fail them in more ways than one, not merely in the substances delivered as medicines, but in the very concept of what medicine is, or should be.

It is beyond a truism in the contemporary UK health landscape that GPs are becoming harder and harder to get to see, and even when we do see them, the encounter can be profoundly unsatisfying. Our governments have become predominantly interested in health as a means of generating wealth for the already wealthy, and in doing so the principles of the UK's National Health Service, free to all at the point of delivery, have been savagely eroded. The evidence for this is an almost daily occurrence in mainstream news reporting. In medicine, as in so many other areas of life, many of us are now feeling strongly that we need to take matters into our own hands.

It is my biggest aspiration for this book that it will contribute materially to the social project of self-empowerment in health and in medicine.

It is, I believe, a project worth fighting for, and my hope is that it, or something very like it, does indeed become the template for future health care in our society, instead of the increasing reliance upon top-down diktats, gold-standard protocols and AI-generated solutions that are in process of engulfing the standard, state-sponsored health offer in most, if not all, of the developed world. We must never forget that we are the punters, the customers: *we tell them what we want, and what is right for us, not the other way around*. We are, after all, paying for it, one way or another,

To advance the cause of Natural Healing and position it where it belongs, at the pinnacle of our understanding of the true dynamics of health and healing, there is a need to give up our reliance on the standard bastions of authority and, with the correct knowledge at our fingertips, take matters into our own hands. This volume is aimed at those who are ready to start that project. I fully understand that some readers will still be largely within the system that we have all inherited from the dominant culture, and that there will need in many cases to be a weaning process. I am not suggesting that you throw your pharmaceuticals into the trash right now—although some may indeed be ready to do that.

In the first instance, if you are dealing with a chronic health problem for which medication of this sort has been prescribed, you need to inform yourself—about the condition, about the treatment, about the possibility of cure, and about your choices. It is not the remit of this book to provide a standard protocol for any named disease that you may have—for a start there are far too many of them, and secondly this is not a professional training manual. That is what we as professional herbalists and natural healers are here for: to help people like you. I did not wake up one day and say, I think I'll go "pharma-free": I saw a lot of practitioners, I learned how to keep myself naturally healthy, and when problems came, I committed to a natural solution *as a first resort*, not, as so often these days, a last-chance crisis effort.

"A herbalist in every home; a practitioner in every community"

For those ready to take the next step, and notwithstanding that you may have tried some of the remedies in this book, I advise that you get yourself a trustworthy, registered natural medicine practitioner. It may cost a bit more than you think you can afford, but it will pay untold dividends, and you will benefit not just from a "treatment", but from a training.

The word *doctor* after all comes from the Latin verb *Docere*—to teach. All natural healers and naturopaths have at the heart of their practice the notion that they are there to impart the methods of self-regulation, not just to act as replacements for your GP. They will teach you things that will be useful, and the gifts that they offer will be the precepts that will inform many years of glowing health and vitality to come. They will also be able to give you specific advice tailored to your individual health profile.

The quotation at the top of this section is again from American herbalist and natural healer Dr John Christopher and represents a manifesto for the School of Natural Healing. It is a template for a decentralised, community-based approach to health care, that leaves no one bereft of help and advice when they need it, at the same time as empowering people in their own homes to take care of simple needs and manage the day-to-day necessities of natural health care.

Dr Christopher's services during his working life were in high demand, and he also frequently travelled some distance to visit and care for his patients, and on that account, he could not necessarily be where he was needed on every occasion, so he made it his business to ensure that the basics were taken care of in the instructions that he left for his patients, as well as to train the next generation of vocational practitioners who would take up the baton in their own service to the communities in which they lived.

In my own practice I frequently declare one of my aims as being to create viable, self-regulating human beings. What I mean by this is that once the "patient" becomes familiar with the methods of self-healing, he begins slowly, or sometimes not so slowly, to achieve independence from patient-hood, and take the first steps towards autonomy in health. This starts with the foundational routines and methods described in this book. These are not specific cures for specific diseases, they are the basis for creating vibrant health and improving your situation wherever you are on the health spectrum. They may not instantly remove your pain and discomfort—this is an unrealistic expectation in the first place, promoted by the purveyors of powerful suppressive medications who would have you believe that the absence of symptoms equates to a cure. But slowly and surely, they will start the process of rebalancing and normalising your physiological processes so that, whatever your starting position, health can begin to prevail.

Incurable people

The other half of Dr Christopher's iteration of the old Avicenna quote: "There are no incurable diseases", was, "... *only incurable people*".

I am not suggesting that there are people who absolutely cannot be "cured". In the first place, no one cures anyone anyway. Nature is the only and ultimate healer for us all and will have her way whatever else we do. What I am saying is that we can, and frequently do, get in the way of our own healing. If we first of all take illness as a necessary message from within to alert us to imbalance and the blocking of vital energy, the next thing we must do is to find, and then address the issue. Our response as individuals to our pain and distress is paramount in determining the outcome. In around 40 years of practice, I have fully learned the truth of the old saying, you can lead a horse to water, but you cannot make him drink.

This is exactly the way it should be. Dr Christopher, whose philosophy is, you will have noticed, somewhat conspicuous in this volume, also gave the advice to practitioners in training, "Do not come until they call." I have to remind students of this time and time again. Do not press-gang your nearest and dearest, your friends, acquaintances and work colleagues, into attending your student clinics. They will agree to come as a favour to you, but if they are not willing to change their default setting when it comes to "medical" interventions, you are both likely to be disappointed. Indeed, their resistance is essential to their own self-determination. Let them know what it is you are doing, be open and informative, but never try to coerce them, or tell them that this *must* be their path. The moment that repeated exposure to your ideas leads to a genuine enquiry, then, possibly, you may have them—at least you have an opening to giving them some practical experience of our methods.

When talking of "cure" it is also necessary to ask, what are we to be cured of? If "disease", or illness, is a natural corrective mechanism, as indeed Natural Healing holds it to be, then there is no cure as such, until the message has been understood and acted upon. Anything else "done to it" is simply marking time, possibly giving some relief, but unlikely to be fully effective until we uncover the deeper significance behind our discomfort.

That is not to say that we may not prevail in rectifying minor ailments with simple remedies, but the deeper, more chronic complaints will demand deeper understanding and a whole body/mind/spirit response that cannot be sidestepped. We must therefore allow our patients, family members, close friends and companions, the freedom to be as they are and to undergo the suffering that is their lot, perhaps acting to soften or reduce the associated pain, but unable to finally and formally remove it for them. The healing is there for all, but it needs full understanding and acceptance on the part of the sufferer.

This may seem a harsh and a tough stance, and you may well disagree vehemently with the sentiment, but without full engagement on the part of the subject of healing, which means full and honest self-examination, working with personal resistance and habit, identifying and recognising the "trip hazards" in our daily lives, results are likely to be at best temporary. While undergoing detoxification, taking the time to nourish the body appropriately, managing the work/rest/play balance, and coming to terms with emotionality and stress, we are also performing work that is focused upon deepening and strengthening our relationship with this "body" that we seem to "have", into a heartfelt and soulful connection with the physical dimension of our greater existence, of which the body is our most intimate reminder.

Living and dying

Someone mischievously said that getting healthy is merely the slowest possible rate at which to die. There is a subtle truth in this. Unless you are a committed immortalist, it is certain that death will catch up with us all at some point. In the quest for perfect health and longevity, this is often forgotten, or maybe we secretly believe we can actually outwit death? We cannot discuss health without enquiring into the nature and purpose of disease, and we cannot talk about life without the awareness of death as the eventual destination.

When it comes to disease and death, we have many value judgments that we mistake for truths: health is good; illness is bad. Life is good, death is bad. The truth is we cannot have one without the other. Without illness, health would have no meaning, and without death, life would be without definition.

My oldest friend in this world died during the writing of this book, at the age of 69—these days considered young indeed. We had known each other from schooldays, aged eleven. He was not particularly interested in health, other than as a means of being able to do the things he wanted to do on this earth, and when he was diagnosed with COPD, he was not in the least bit inclined to give up his beloved cigarettes.

He died peacefully one afternoon in his back garden, smoking a cigarette and drinking a cup of strong black coffee. When news of his death reached me, apart from the poignant sense of personal loss, that we would never again hang out together and reminisce, put the world to rights, lambast our common enemies and *bêtes noirs*, I was also struck by the perfection of his death, and I knew that it was both timely and fitting, and that he would have been pleased enough by it. I knew that he had done what he needed to do here, and there was no reason to stay. Granted, he was single with no heirs and few close relatives. He had organised a direct cremation, no ceremony, no "remembrance" service. I knew he did not need that. And neither did I. He lives on in my experience as vitally now as when he was alive, and almost every day I experience the gratitude of having known him.

Naturopath Andreas Moritz, who discovered and wrote *The Amazing Liver and Gallbladder Flush*[12] (mentioned in Chapter 3) died in 2012 at the age of 58. Many people took that as a signal that the methods he spent his life espousing and teaching were ineffective—but they wrote their unkind evaluations in ignorance of the fact that Andreas was diagnosed with juvenile rheumatoid arthritis and cardiac arrhythmia in early childhood, and not expected to live much beyond his teen years. A life spent staying alive using natural healing techniques is hardly wasted, and to outlive one's prognosis by nearly 40 years an achievement in itself.

The message is, although we clearly prize quantity where life expectancy is concerned, quality and achievement are arguably more important. No one wants to die, but death will catch up with us all eventually. The ways in which we ready ourselves for that are as numerous as we are, I suspect, and some may never be ready. This is maybe not the place to talk about the metaphysical implications of these statements: I leave you to your own beliefs in that respect. But most would agree that quality of life to the end, over quantity at any cost, is preferable, and there is in the end no one who can evaluate this other than each one of us for ourselves.

The spectrum of wellness

The spectrum of wellness is a teaching tool that I have developed for classroom use. It consists of a simple diagram involving a horizontal line. At one end of the line—say the right-hand end—we are as fully and vibrantly alive as it is possible to be. At the other end we are...dead.

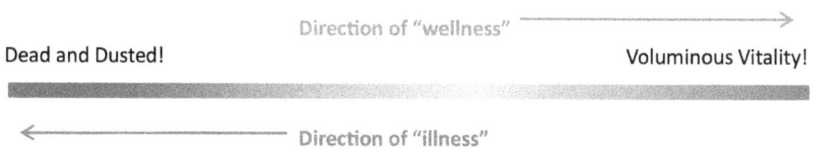

Figure 8. The spectrum of wellness.

Most of us spend our time somewhere in the middle, some closer to health, some closer to illness, but the most fundamental truth about this situation is that it is <u>completely changeable and open to influence</u>. In fact is always in a dynamic state of flux. It may be influenced by factors operating in the external environment, by "stress", by our own chosen lifestyle habits, and by our psychological and emotional settings.

Some will by now have intuitively realised that this is nothing more nor less than a reiteration of the theory outlined in Chapter 1 and points to the deployment of methods espoused in the doctrine of the *Six Non-Naturals*, as expounded in detail over Chapters 2 to 7. So, I am not saying anything new here, but I am unapologetically reiterating the central message:

YOU CAN MAKE A DIFFERENCE!

In fact, ONLY YOU can make a difference. It is your actions, choices, preferences and beliefs concerning health that have the power to change the direction of those arrows in the diagram and move yourself either towards illness (and death) or towards abundant vitality and health. And the only way you are going to be able to verify this is by doing it. If health is your preferred direction, start implementing the advice in this book now.

You don't have to do it all at once: choose one or two areas in which you would like to work—maybe your diet and eating patterns, or your choice of household products. When these changes have become habitual, focus on the next phase—maybe you'd like to give some simple detoxification programmes a try? Maybe setting up an exercise plan that is achievable for you?

To assist you I have included a sample Natural Healing Implementation Template at the end of this chapter, referenced to the individual chapters in this book. Whatever you do, if you are currently in relatively good health and you want to preserve that situation for as long as possible, START NOW, in whatever way is appropriate for you.

At all points you are in control—it is your life, your programme. You always have the option to take advice—that is what practitioners like me are here for. You may also find webinars and workshops given by some of us beneficial. I'll only put one caution in your way here: in every case check out what is being offered with the Natural Healing Filter firmly in the "ON" position. There are plenty of "virgin sex counsellors" out there (think about that one!). Testimonials are always advisable from those who have benefited from the advice they give, but they must not necessarily replace your own intuition and judgement, and if necessary, ask the difficult questions before you take on anyone else's advice. Hopefully reading this book will have already started to hone your skills of discrimination and evaluation.

Here is a template for a simple health checklist that you can draw up to begin to plan your Natural Healing journey:

Topic	What you are currently doing that helps?	What you are currently doing that hinders?	What do you need to put in place to improve?	Chapter/ comments
Detoxification				Chapters 2 & 3
Food and Drink				Chapter 4
Ambient Air				Chapter 5
Movement and Rest				Chapter 6
Perturbations of Mind and Spirit				Chapter 7
Creating the healing space, working with beliefs				Chapters 9 & 10

Figure 9. Personal health plan check list.

Endnotes

1. Foucault, M. (2003). *The Birth of the Clinic* (London & New York: Routledge).
2. UK Government (2024). *What is the WHO Pandemic Preparedness Treaty?* https://commonslibrary.parliament.uk/research-briefings/cbp-9550/.

3. Jackson, T. (2025). *The Care Economy*. Cambridge: Polity.
4. https://www.independent.co.uk/tv/news/noam-chomsky-calls-for-unvaccinated-to-be-isolated-from-society-b2182947.html.
5. https://www.who.int/news-room/questions-and-answers/item/herd-immunity-lockdowns-and-covid-19.
6. For more detail on these statements read: Trebing, W. P. (2019). *Good-Bye Germ Theory*. Author.
7. Simian vacuolating virus (SV40) was a component of the original polio vaccine, and was controversially implicated in carcinogenesis. This vaccine was replaced in 1965 by the Salk vaccine, but "fragments" of the virus have since surfaced as "starting material" in other vaccines, notably the Pfizer MRNA Covid-19 jab. Needless to say the official narrative is that it is inert and safe, but not all physicians agree: see https://www.infectioncontroltoday.com/view/florida-surgeon-general-raises-concerns-over-dna-contaminants-pfizer-and-moderna-covid-19-vaccines.
8. https://pmc.ncbi.nlm.nih.gov/articles/PMC7515561/.
9. Mendelsohn, R.S. (1979). *Confessions of a Medical Heretic* (New York: McGraw-Hill).
10. Read Goldacre, B. (2013). *Bad Pharma: How Medicine is Broken, and How We Can Fix It* (London, 4th Estate).
11. Wardle, J., Steel, A., Lauche, R. & Adams, J. (2017). Collaborating with Medicine? Perceptions of Australian Naturopaths on Integrating within the Conventional Medical System. *Journal of Interprofessional Care* 31(6): 734–743. Retrieved from: http://www.tandfonline.com/doi/full/10.1080/13561820.2017.1351424.
12. Moritz, A. (2012). *The Amazing Liver and Gallbladder Flush* (ebook: Ener-chi.com).

CHAPTER TEN

The space of healing

In order to heal, we need to be able to create a healing environment. This is not just candles and incense—although for some these paraphernalia are helpful in focusing energy towards healing—but also a space *within ourselves* wherein we might begin to apprehend and make contact with that powerful, non-local, quantum energy that we have called the Vital Force, or the Healing Power of Nature. This chapter is about how we can create that space in our very minds, wherever we are, and whatever we are doing.

In order to activate this there are two areas in which we need to focus our attention. One is towards our beliefs concerning health and healing. The other is the ability to switch into what I call *The Space of Healing*, at any time we choose. In both endeavours it is the content of our mind that concerns us. This is not just "positive thinking": we can accept the probability that our minds will occasionally generate negative and fearful thoughts and feelings; but it is the possibility that we do not necessarily have to remain with those effects that perhaps we can begin to grasp, and towards which we can direct some self-entrainment.

Again, we are not talking about a suppressive practice here, where we affirm the "positive" over the "negative": in any case, as natural healers we do not necessarily regard symptoms as "negative", they are simply communications from within. We will look at affirmations later in this chapter, and in particular we will explore a way of working with positive suggestions, using them in a diagnostic capacity in order to gain more knowledge about ourselves and our fundamental beliefs. However as someone once pointed out, repeating affirmations can be a bit like going into your garden with your eyes tight shut and saying over and over, "There are no weeds in my garden, there are no weeds in my garden …", and then being disappointed on opening your eyes to see that there are in fact still plenty of weeds! (And weeds, as herbalists well know, are often powerful healers in their own right).

To start <u>where we are</u>, not from some imagined point of perfection, is simply realistic, and the perspective that where we are is also, in its own way, *perfect*, is an act of faith in itself—faith that we can, from whichever starting point, influence the situation and prevail in changing it, should that be the most desirable outcome. As we will see, you cannot make a fool of the mind: it is there to protect your psychological integrity, to make sense of the world it perceives, and to ensure that you are not caught in a contradiction. Your beliefs have been carefully selected to chime in with your culture, your personality and your life-purpose. However, they can be changed if they are found to be inhibiting your progress—or making you sick!

The critical importance of health beliefs

Remember Dr Christopher's famous saying, "There are no incurable diseases, only incurable people"? One of the ways to render yourself incurable is to *believe* that you are incurable. If you start a healing journey already secretly convinced that it is not possible, then guess what? It won't be—that is, not until you change that belief. The rule is that the body will never contradict the inner convictions of the mind. If it did we would be in a permanent state of cognitive dissonance.

This is often the biggest hurdle to be overcome, particularly in those who have received a diagnosis of "incurability", because not only have we all been brought up to believe that some things are just not possible, but also, when that is reinforced by the authority of medical opinion, it can become an immovable object.

In my own struggle with my hip my first instinct was no different from my approach to anything else, but the more I sought help (including, as mentioned above, from natural medicine practitioners), the more convinced I became of the official, conventional view of my situation. In the absence of verifiable "cures" without surgery (and excepting stem-cell treatment, which even if I wanted to go there I could not afford), I concluded somewhat painfully that I was deluded in thinking I could change the prognosis, and that it was time to come to terms with the "reality" of my situation, as so many people were describing it to me. I began to look for accredited and recommended orthopaedic surgeons.

It can certainly happen that the people around you will, peculiarly, instead of encouraging you to proceed according to your own convictions, berate and scold you, and try to get you to take the path *they* feel is appropriate. In most cases this is well-meaning—although my next door neighbour did call me a "bloody idiot" when I told him I was not going to get the surgery—but it can have serious consequences. In the case of cancer, for example, I have seen those who set out, with my help or that of other suitably trained and experienced practitioners, upon a path of Natural Healing, are subjected to so much negativity and fear coming at them from their family and friends that they frequently find it easier to give up the attempt and capitulate to the orthodoxy.

In my case I was fortunate enough to have family around me who fully supported my choices. My son, in particular, listening to me one day fretting about whether I should get myself booked into the medical system for a hip replacement, finally said, "Look dad, you've spent your whole life working in the field of natural medicine. You've been trained by some of the best. Why give up now? You *know* you can beat this!" Having himself been trained in methods of improving levels of strength and suppleness of the musculoskeletal system, he also shared some specific exercises with me, and to my astonishment I noticed almost immediate improvements.

To explain my near-capitulation, it is necessary to understand that hip arthritis is extremely and continuously painful, debilitating, depressing and demoralising. Knowing as I now do how chronic pain can erode and sap one's vitality and focus has given me an intimate understanding of the issues around belief and dedication to the path of healing.

I did a lot of things supposedly correctly. I had tried several "natural" remedies and experienced very little improvement, and in fact an overall worsening over time. For example, for many months I took high-dose curcumin supplements, sometimes blended with other herbs for which clinical evidence exists in the case of severe arthritis. My diet was basically sound, and I knew the foods that I needed, according to nutritionists, to avoid. I exercised as much as I could within the limitations of my condition, and I sought help from physical therapists. There is nothing more belief-sapping that when the things you believe in are obviously failing you.

But what I eventually realised was that my focus was wrong. I was using natural supplements—herbal extracts—*as though they were pharmaceuticals*, for their "anti-inflammatory" properties. Curcumin, for example, had scored well against ibuprofen in trials for the relief of arthritic pain. Curcuma itself—the plant Turmeric—is much more than an anti-inflammatory, of course, and curcumin is an example of the use of an isolated plant extract in place of the whole plant, chosen specifically to suppress inflammation and "kill pain". It was a schoolboy error, and one that I could scarcely believe of myself at the moment of realisation. With the benefit of hindsight I am inclined to take a more lenient view: I had never been subjected to that much ongoing pain and disability in my life, and the messages I was getting almost everywhere I looked were, quite explicitly, focused on the incurability of my condition. Despite my familiarity with Dr Christopher's famous statement on the matter, I missed the fact that I was drifting away from my own principles.

I decided to shift focus, and reinforce the *belief* that I could find a solution. I had found no externally validated evidence of or testimony to non-surgical cures in conditions similar to mine, hence in my mind I had to become a pioneer. I immediately felt more empowered, and I redoubled my research efforts, while simultaneously working on the underlying beliefs and emotions concerning my problem. If I found myself entertaining doubt about the outcome I would remind myself that failure was not an option. What was it that Thomas Edison reputedly said when challenged that it took him 7000 attempts to make a lightbulb? "Actually, I received 6999 lessons in how NOT to make a lightbulb."

Recognising and changing up when things are not working is essential, in the same way that we discussed earlier in terms of clearing the space of old debris so that new health could be built in its place. It's the same with beliefs. You need to clear out the ones that do not serve—but first you have to find them, and they can be tricky. They can hide; but there are ways to bring them to consciousness. For the avoidance of misunderstanding, I am not saying here that belief in itself will do the trick. I am saying that it is necessary to adopt commensurate beliefs in order to activate your best efforts at solving the problem.

Take Avicenna's framing of the now-oft-repeated adage: "*There are no incurable diseases; only the want of knowledge.*" You have to believe the first proposition in order to be able to benefit from the second. If you believe that your disease is incurable you are unlikely to look very hard for the means of curing it.

However, positive though it is to start by implanting a helpful belief, it also needs to be nourished and watered in an appropriate soil—the soil of your overall world view. If your world view is heavily influenced by what we might call an "objectivist paradigm"—that is to say, a thing is either objectively true or it isn't, and you can't change it—then your new belief in curability is going to have a hard time growing mature enough to bear fruit. You are going to need to do some more work on that.

For example, you could remind yourself that the lessons of the past strongly suggest that what science, or medicine, believes is true in one era is often proved false in a future era. You can find endless examples of this in the history of science. How about the ridicule that Robert Stephenson was subjected to when he proposed that would build a means of transport that would run on tracks at speeds of up to forty miles an hour? They said it couldn't be done because the passengers would fall off. The more ridiculous the example the better for your case. Medical history is also full of examples of things that could not be done but have been proven to be possible—regeneration of brain and nerve cells, for example.

In my case this applied to cartilage. I came across a study that suggested that the availability of stem cells for cartilage repair differed according to location in the body. Apparently there are plenty in the ankle, fewer in the knee, and fewer still in the hip, and that is why hip arthritis does not repair naturally. This is the idea behind stem-cell therapy, where cells are injected into the hip joint to stimulate cartilage growth (the treatment is not available on the NHS and is very expensive). But the thought that occurred to me was, "Aha, so there may not be that *many*, but there are *some*: how can we get those activated? Or how can we promote higher levels in that location?" This immediately started to generate results that, had I stopped with, "It can't be done", would not have been visible.

For me the real meaning of Natural Healing, and the most fundamental belief necessary for healing, is as simple as this:

The body repairs itself

We could add, "Using the vital energy with which we are all endowed by Nature, and *if we take appropriate measures to create the right conditions*." This will not apply in extreme cases: if you lose a limb or an organ it will generally not regrow; but in most cases of ordinary wear and tear, injury as a result of disturbances of homeostasis, and trauma that is not destructive of the basic given structure, repair is possible. As Swiss naturopath and herbalist Alfred Vogel said, *"Whatever disease the body has produced, it is able to reverse."*

Where it does not happen, two main mechanisms apply:

1. The conditions are not right to promote the self-healing.
2. There is a deeper meaning behind the symptom that needs to be uncovered and worked with.

In case of reason number 1, the advice given in the foregoing pages of this book serves to provide reliable methods of activating this innate self-healing mechanism. In the case of reason number 2, the most common prohibition stems from doubt and disbelief. Your body will always faithfully reproduce your expectations and beliefs. In this case, the work that needs to be done in order to activate the healing is the conscientious examination of those beliefs, where they came from, and the emotions invested in them. Additional advice concerning difficult or negative emotions is given in Chapter 7, but my previous book, *The Mind's Eye*, is also largely dedicated to this topic.

There is no more powerful belief that you can have in relation to your health, than that your body knows how to heal itself, and that you can consciously and directly promote and potentiate that ability. Therefore ensure that you are diligent in seeking out and identifying any lingering doubts, prevarications, conditional asides and accommodations that you may be harbouring: "Yes I believe *in theory* that my body will heal itself, but in my case there are special reasons why this won't necessarily happen."

Behind this there may be other beliefs that are far more personal and insidious, such as, "I would commit to healing myself but actually

I deserve to be ill," or "I need to be ill in order to learn certain lessons, atone for certain other shortcomings (or *Karma*), of because illness is somehow a necessity in life that I cannot (should not) avoid." There are many versions of these beliefs—take your pick, and learn to tune into your own personal versions, and observe the twists and turns of your own mind as you seek to bring them to the light of day.

Affirmations

Affirmations can be helpful, but they do need to be carefully constructed and diligently monitored. If for example you want to attract wealth, but you have a belief that rich people are only rich at the expense of poor people, you may not succeed, as you will not want to be a member of that club. If you want to heal and be healthy, but you don't want to have to do the supporting work, you may find that your health is short-lived or superficial, or that the problem you have chosen to focus on does indeed resolve, only to be replaced by a bigger one further down the line.

In each case the underlying beliefs, and the "core beliefs" (a "core belief" is a belief that may underlie your view of the world but often remains hidden because it is so obvious that you cannot distinguish it from "reality"), will, if contradictory to the belief you want to establish, interrupt the flow of energy to the desired outcome. Examples here—and they are extreme—are beliefs about the fundamental nature of the world and appearances: you cannot walk through walls because walls are solid—you can try but you will hurt yourself; you cannot shapeshift into another animal because your DNA is human. Nevertheless there are places in the world where people believe that both these things may be achieved, *and in their terms*, they are fully realisable.

An example of a core belief that affects a good many people in the developed world is that healing is only achieved through the use of drugs and substances, and that nothing exists other than physical substance. Your body, for instance, is purely physical substance, and therefore will respond, mechanistically, to the introduction of other physical substances that are designed to change its state. In that context, the proposition that medicines may have "vibrational" or "energetic" effects, or be more than simply physical substance, is the purest idiocy and a classic example of "pseudoscience".

If this forms a core belief in your system you will have trouble believing in the "healing power of nature", for sure, and you may therefore tend to place a high premium on the opinions of doctors who have been trained in "objectivist" science.

At the opposite end of the spectrum of belief is the religious notion that illness is visited upon us by a punitive god, or gods, and that in order to heal we must learn to propitiate that entity in whatever way he/she/it demands. In this case also, the possibility of healing is diminished, as the balance of power is once again with something external to you.

However, if you are inclined to believe that we don't necessarily know all there is to know about reality, then you are likely to have an open mind, and can work very effectively with the tool of affirmation. Here is a "conversation" that you might have with yourself along the lines of attempting to establish a working belief in the possibility of healing: in the exchange below, the "response" is your own inner voice, offering its objections, and thus of course revealing the underlying beliefs that maybe in some cases you didn't know you held.

Affirmation:	*My body knows how to heal itself to perfection.*
Response:	*Yes, but ... its ability to do so is limited. Doctors are not stupid people, they'd know if it were possible to heal what I've got.*
Revised affirmation:	*My body has unlimited powers of self-healing.*
Response:	*OK, but what if the doctors are right, and I am wrong?*
Revised affirmation:	*My beliefs are powerful: they shape my reality. I choose to believe in my powers of healing.*
Response:	*Ah, but maybe it's not OK for me to heal myself? Maybe there's a reason why I am ill. Maybe I deserve to be ill?* (notice how the inner voice skips onto a different track here—you are getting closer to the real reason for your difficulty in believing in your self-healing abilities).
Revised affirmation:	*I deserve to be fully and vitally alive and well. I believe in my own essential goodness, and in the goodness of the universe.*

Notice how the revised affirmations never grapple with the negativity of the response or seek to suppress that belief: they simply insert a positive statement that you can then choose to adopt instead. The truth about belief is that it is possibly the most powerful tool we possess in pursuit of our own healing. Belief is literally constitutional, but your system, your consciousness, will never let itself be made a fool of. If you try and believe something that is against a deeper belief that you have, it will not allow the new belief to be successful—until you also change the pre-eminent belief. If you are ready to go to the sublimest levels, however, here is a beautiful healing affirmation that I have used to excellent effect many times:

*Every cell in my body is bathed perpetually
in the radiance of my divine being.*

There is one more vital perspective to impart here. <u>Investment in your belief in the self-healing capacity of your body needs to be matched by withdrawal of the energy directed towards maintaining the awareness of illness.</u> This may seem counter-intuitive, especially when we are also advocating the theory that illness functions as a wake-up call. However, reinforcing that we ARE ill, that we HAVE such and such a condition, serves to compound and perpetuate the condition itself. Even the simple acquisition of a diagnosis can do this: as soon as you fix the illness into a specific condition, you reinforce the idea that this is now a part of you, and you build it ever more concretely into your idea of who and what you are. In this way, even directing your thoughts into "fighting illness" (as opposed to creating health) serves to reinforce the illness. As Newton famously observed, every action is automatically met by an equal and opposite reaction, and an obvious consequence of fighting illness is that it may fight back!

In all of this, awareness of language, and the use of language, is paramount. The verb "to spell" has a double meaning: it is only partly about the correct order of letters in a word. The rest of it is about the "spell" that is cast by language in creating, defining and maintaining your reality. Try to avoid "spellbinding" yourself by reinforcing the idea of illness as an objective condition.

Instead, focus on "illness" as a configuration of energy, labile and flexible, ever-changing (like the arrows in the spectrum of wellness discussed in Chapter 9) and open to easy influence. The following are offered as a set of basic suggestions for managing your awareness of illness.

- Do not OWN your illness: do not say "I HAVE asthma", or "I AM asthmatic". Say rather, my chest needs to relax now, or my airways need space to open.
- Affirm the ability of your body to respond to these suggestions. As time goes on you will be able to offer these statements as positive intentions for your body: "My airways are now free to open fully".

- If you are experiencing pain, you can use this method to turn it off, but only if you are also conscientiously working to restore the basic harmony of the body.
- In this case the suggestion would be something like: "It's OK to stop sending me these signals for the time being: I have received and understood the message".
- If you are aware that conditions around you are exacerbating a feeling of illness, do what you can to step away from them or counteract them. Affirm your willingness to give your body the space to heal.

The space of healing

I was being treated by my osteopath and she observed that I had, as she thought, "fallen asleep": I replied no, I had been conscious all the way through, but that I was in an altered state of reality, a very deep and relaxed state, in which I could strongly feel the energy in my body working to heal itself, directed and unblocked by her treatment.

She said, "That's the space of healing," and I suddenly realised, she's right. There is a specific state of consciousness that can facilitate healing, and it is somewhat recognisable, although you may not know what is truly possible within it. Many readers will be familiar with it. We might access it almost by accident, in a reverie in nature, or simply in front of the fire on a dark winter's afternoon, after a warm bath lying relaxing on your bed, on a long train journey with nothing to do except daydream. To some extent it is similar to the "hypnogogic" state we sometimes attain before falling sleep; indeed it is possible to use the pre-sleep state to insert healing suggestions that your body can act upon while in the sleep state.

Healing will not take place in the context of fear and anxiety. This is one of the shortcomings of our typical response to illness and injury. Fear is a physiological state of constriction and heightened adrenal vigilance. Healing needs expansion and relaxation. We might say it's similar to the difference between sympathetic and parasympathetic nerve responses, except that it is perfectly possible to be in a sympathetic state and also to be positive and constructive. For example, the physiological state of fear and panic is rather similar to that of excitement: increased heart-rate, dilation of pupils, palmar sweating, hyperventilation and so forth. On the one hand, however, the *interpretation* of these sensations and phenomena goes towards risk and danger, and on the other hand towards the thrill of an enjoyable activity. Performers are well aware of the knife-edge between stage-fright, and being pumped and "in the zone". Some indeed welcome risk and danger as an enjoyable experience.

It is also possible to be both "relaxed" (or unmotivated) and depressed and worried, and this again will not lead to healing. It is a simple formulation, but you have to put positive emotions into the mix: love, joy, hope, excitement. The key to manifesting anything, including vibrant, powerful health, is to hold your intended goal in mind (what you want or need to heal in yourself), mix it up with one of these emotions, and then just relax in the certain knowledge that you have already created it. I recommend a practice of just 10 minutes a day with this formula. No more; don't overdo it or it may become obsession, which flips into the anxiety state. Here is the exercise in full:

- Find a comfortable space in which to sit or lie, and feel yourself as relaxed as possible.
- Have a clear intention in mind—a health goal, in our terms here. You can make it a general goal, but if you have a few different issues, then choose just one to work with.
- Visualise yourself fully healed, recovered, no longer experiencing this issue—pain, symptom or diagnosis.
- With that image clearly in mind, call up a powerful, positive emotion—love, joy, gratitude, hope, excitement. It can help to realise that these emotions usually centre in or around the heart—they are *heartfelt*. If you cannot make contact with any such emotions, then try and recall a moment in your life when you did experience a similar emotion and "import" that into your current situation.
- Remain in that space for a few minutes only, and then affirm to yourself that your ideal outcome has already been created and is waiting for you.

Do not get demoralised if results are not instant. In a quantum, time-collapsed state, they have indeed already been actioned. Things move at a slower vibrational rate on the physical plane, and we need to wait for them to catch up with the intention we have already created. We also need time to do the "legwork" on the physical plane—the active pursuit of a natural lifestyle that will be an important part of the mechanism of delivery.

An over-concern with fatigue, emotional or physical, is understandable, but again unproductive. Instead of complaining about how tired you are, simply give yourself full and joyful permission to rest, and then instruct the body that now is the time to refresh, regenerate and revive itself. If you find yourself unable to relax and rest, ask yourself why? Often the answer will present as some obligation or the sense of "a million and one things to do", or some other cause of ongoing anxiety.

The Neurogenic iris types (Iridology disposition)[1] among us are particularly good at keeping themselves on the go long after they really should have stopped. Neurogenics live on their nerves, and they are programmed to believe that the world will grind to a halt if they are not there to keep it spinning around. Consequently they are more prone than most to "burn out", no matter that they also nominally possess above-average constitutional strength.

It is a matter of putting yourself in charge of yourself and your life, and refusing to hand that responsibility over to anyone or anything else. Looking after yourself is not selfish, it is necessary. I often remind our neurogenic brothers and sisters that they will certainly not be able to fulfil their (often self-imposed) raft of obligations once they have finally and officially driven themselves into the ground (or even six feet under!). Learning the art of pacing yourself, prioritising what really needs to be done and relegating what does not—or scheduling it for a later opportunity—is a highly necessary life-skill in our fast-paced, manic world.

Again, some of our cherished cultural tropes may work against us here: the saying, "Procrastination is the thief of time," which first appeared in a poem by the English poet Edward Young (1683–1765), has been taken out of context as a prohibition against ever putting anything off to a later date. Instead, the inverted version, "Never do today what you can usefully put off till tomorrow," will occasionally serve well—but only as long as you can also allay any tendency to worry about it!

Your compulsive busyness might be a response to the idea, inserted when you were quite young, that you have to be "perfect", or perform in some particular way, in order to deserve life's rewards. In this case it is worth reminding yourself that you are now in command of your own life, and it is for no one but yourself to determine the rhythms and cycles that enable you to establish a state of grace and favour in your life. This is a powerful position to take, as it affirms your sovereignty over your body and over your life: *choose* to do the things you do, but do not allow yourself to be *compelled* into doing them.

Time to heal

As well as space, healing also needs to be given time. Once upon a time people used to be expected to take a period of convalescence after an illness, or a surgical procedure. The word comes from the Latin *valescere*—to grow strong; convalesce—*to grow strong with*.

You may well have noticed that the ideal situation in medicine these days is to shorten the recovery period as much as possible. When I had an appendectomy in 1966 I was hospitalised for 2 weeks: these days children typically go home 24 to 36 hours after the surgery. That's not to say that home may not be the best place, or that these children are not also accorded a period of rest and absence from school, but I look back fondly on my hospitalisation as a holiday from my busy family home where my parents were also bringing up four other children (at that time—soon to be five) in the midst of a busy work schedule. Different horizons, spending time being wheeled around the beautiful grounds of Carshalton children's hospital, nurses who were fun to talk to and play with, other children who were also undergoing treatment, camaraderie and conviviality in healing. I wept when I had to leave—much to the annoyance of my parents.

The time that is necessary to heal is not just a function of the rate of physical healing; it is also related to the need for psychological and emotional readjustment, and perhaps even re-evaluation. To hurry the healing process, and then dive straight back into a lifestyle that was probably at least partly responsible for making you sick in the first place, is a fast track to becoming sick again very quickly. The adjustments that may need to take place are not merely physical: emotional learning and integration also needs to take place, and for this a rest from ordinary activity is crucial.

I could also point out that if you give yourself time for healing and regeneration within the structure of your normal life you might not get so sick in the first place, but it is easy to be wise in retrospect—it was German naturopath and historian of Nature Cure, Alfred Brauchle (1898–1964), who reputedly said, "Only those whose lives are threatened take up nature cure." This is something that we often observe in practice: patients will present only after conventional routes of treatment have been explored and found wanting, and when the situation is at its most dire. At that point the journey to reverse the process is necessarily a long one, and it cannot be rushed.

The central message here is that ALL illness calls upon us to consider what we might need to do differently, in order to live closer to Nature, but also closer to our own truth. There are several narratives that suggest that the call of the future—our future selves calling to us down the years to become more of who we are, perhaps—is a more powerful rationale for illness than the "sins" and mistakes of the past.

In *The Healing Power of Illness*[2] Thorwald Dethelfsen and Rüdiger Dalhke suggest that illness calls its own resolution into being, which is necessarily in the future; and in Doug Boyd's book, the eponymous hero, Native American medicine man Rolling Thunder,[3] had his patients meditate for three days on what they would do with their health once regained, before he would accept them for healing. We don't just get well because illness isn't very nice and we deserve to get better: we get well because we need to fulfil our mission here on earth. And, as Richard Bach[4] suggested, "There is no such thing as a problem without a gift for you in its hands; we seek problems because we need their gifts."

The miracle of life

The gift of healing is our birthright, but we have to come forward to claim it. I hope that this book goes some way towards providing a road map for those who wish to step up to the challenge. This is not to suggest that miracles may not happen, with or without all the seeming "hard work" and privation—the giving up of favourite foods and cherished habits, the punishing exercise and cold water routines, the purging of the detox protocols.

Healing is indeed a miracle, whenever and however it happens. It is the miracle of life itself, in all of its full and fantastic potential, across aeons of time and multifarious dimensions of existence. Healing affirms our essential nature as children of the universe, divine and blessed—even if we do not believe that that is who we are.

I wish every reader joy and success in following their individual path to freedom in health and vitality. Believe in yourselves, in Nature—the Nature that is in you, and in us all, the Nature that you *are*—and in your unique journey, and then bear witness to what you, uniquely, know to be true. Every journey, every success and triumph, every *healing*, enriches us all, and shows us the way when we are faltering, in moments of darkness and doubt, when we need a hand to hold, when we feel furthest away from the grace that we crave. Because the truth is that the power and ability to heal is inside each and every one of us.

We are alive, and everything may be achieved.[5]

Endnotes

1. My previous book, *Practical Iridology*, discusses these physiological types in terms of behaviour and typical responses to stress and busyness; it is worth taking the time to discover and understand your type.
2. Thorwald, D. & Dahlke, R. (1995). *The Healing Power of Illness* (London: Element).
3. Boyd, D. (1976). *Rolling Thunder* (London: Bantam Doubleday Dell).
4. Bach, R. (1998). *Illusions: The Adventures of a Reluctant Messiah* (London: Arrow).
5. Bhabra, H.S. (1986). *Gestures* (London: Michael Joseph), p. 73.

ACKNOWLEDGMENTS

Profound thanks are due to my wife and partner in all things meaningful, Anji Main, who has shared my journey in almost every detail, and who has been the best partner I could have wished for in my peculiar *Arbeitslauf/Lebenslauf*. Her presence in these pages is constitutional and unmissable.

To my mother, Valerie, with whom I shared a lively interest in "the alternatives" from an early age. I remember especially sitting watching "Yoga with Richard Hittleman" with her in an early incarnation of daytime TV when I was around 15, and attending with her the very first *Mind, Body Spirit* festival in the Royal Horticultural Halls in 1977 (Subsequently I have become a regular exhibitor at this show).

To my father, Richard, who deserves to be, as he used to tell us he would be, the "King of the World", for his unabashed admixture of the scientific and the spiritual.

To my son, Aaron, who has taught me more things than he realises, and whose incisive critiques of my world I have learned to trust as embodiments of the sword of Manjushri.

To my daughter (in all but the biological sense) Chloe, who is herself an intuitive natural healer, and a true crusader for sovereignty in health and self-determination.

To my teachers, both here and hereafter, without whom none of this might have happened.

To the Vital Force itself, the *Vis Medicatrix Naturae*, that ineffable component of us all which constantly sustains and nourishes.

BIBLIOGRAPHY

Alasfar, R. & Isaifan, R. (2021). Aluminum Environmental Pollution: The Silent Killer. *Environmental Science and Pollution Research*, 28(33): 44587–44597. Available at: https://pmc.ncbi.nlm.nih.gov/articles/PMC8364537/

Anderson, J. & Abrahamson, K. (2017). Your Health Care May Kill You: Medical Errors. *Studies in Health Technology and Informatics*, 234: 13–17. Available at: https://pubmed.ncbi.nlm.nih.gov/28186008/

Anonymous. (n.d.). *Background and Environmental Exposures to Aluminum in the United States.* Available at: https://www.atsdr.cdc.gov/toxprofiles/tp22-c2.pdf

Bach, E. (2005). *The Essential Writings of Dr Edward Bach: The Twelve Healers and Heal Thyself.* London: Vermilion.

Bach, R. (1998). *Illusions: The Adventures of a Reluctant Messiah.* London: Arrow.

Batmangelidj, F. (2008). *Your Body's Many Cries for Water.* Falls Church: Global Health Solutions.

BBC. (n.d.). *Tackling Climate Change with Technology.* Available at: http://news.bbc.co.uk/1/hi/technology/8338853.stm

Bhabra, H.S. (1986). *Gestures.* London: Michael Joseph.

Bone, K. (n.d.). *Echinacea: A New Perspective on its Benefits*. Available at: https://www.naturopathy-uk.com/news/news-cnm-blog/blog/2018/09/26/echinacea-root-a-new-perspective-on-its-benefits/
Boyd, D. (1976). *Rolling Thunder*. New York: Bantam Doubleday Dell.
Bryson, C. (2006). *The Fluoride Deception*. New York: Seven Stories Press.
Buettner, D. (2023). *The Blue Zones: Secrets for Living Longer*. Washington, DC: National Geographic.
Burroughs, S. (2019). *The Master Cleanser*. London: Albatross Publishers.
Campbell, P. (2022). *Eat Right, Lose Weight*. London: Lagom.
Campbell, T.C. & Campbell, M. (2017). *The China Study: Revised and Expanded Edition*. Dallas: BenBella Books.
Cannon, W. (1963). *The Wisdom of the Body*. New York: W. W. Norton and Company Inc.
Christopher, D. (1993). *An Herbal Legacy of Courage*. Springville: Christopher Publications.
Christopher, J.R. (2019). *The School of Natural Healing*. Springville: Christopher Publications.
Christopher, J.R. (2014). *Herbal Home Health Care*. Springville: Christopher Publications.
Christopher, J.R. (1991). *Curing the Incurables*. Springville: Christopher Enterprises.
Cohen, A. (2021). *A Bill Gates Venture Aims To Spray Dust Into The Atmosphere To Block The Sun. What Could Go Wrong*? Available at: https://www.forbes.com/sites/arielcohen/2021/01/11/bill-gates-backed-climate-solution-gains-traction-but-concerns-linger/
Cowan, T. & Fallon, S. (2020). *The Contagion Myth: Why Viruses (including "Coronavirus") Are Not the Cause of Disease*. Oxford: Blackwell.
Crops not Shops, Sustainable Food and Community Growing Project. (n.d.). https://www.cropsnotshops.co.uk
D'Adamo, P. (1997). *Eat Right 4 Your Type*. New York: Berkley.
De Baïracli Levy, J. (1970). *The Natural Rearing of Children*. London: Faber & Faber.
Deruelle, F. (2021). Are Persistent Aircraft Trails a Threat to the Environment and to Health? *Reviews on Environmental Health*, 37(3): 407–421. Available at: https://doi.org/10.1515/reveh-2021-0060
Dethlefsen, T. & Dahlke, R. (1995). *The Healing Power of Illness*. London: Element.
Diamond, H. & Diamond, M. (1987). *Fit for Life*. New York: Bantam.
Dincin Buchman, D. (1995). *The Complete Book of Water Therapy*. New York: McGraw Hill Education.
Dispenza, J. (2014). *You are the Placebo: Making your Mind Matter*. London: Hay House.

Doolittle, W.F. (2013). Microbial Neopleomorphism. *Biology and Philosophy*, 28(2): 351–378. https://doi.org/10.1007/s10539-012-9358-7

Evans, P., Hucklebridge, F. & Clow, A. (2000), *Mind, Immunity and Health: The Science of Psychoneuroimmunology*. London: Free Association Books.

Fennell, J. (2002). *The Dog Listener: Learning the Language of Your Best Friend*. London: HarperCollins.

Foucault, M. (2003). *The Birth of the Clinic*. London & New York: Routledge.

Ghirga, G. (2022). Who Cares About Climate Change? *BMJ*, 377: o1150. doi: https://doi.org/10.1136/bmj.o1150

Goldacre, B. (2013). *Bad Pharma: How Medicine is Broken, and How We Can Fix It*. London: 4th Estate.

Harrison, J. (2018). *Love Your Disease: It's Keeping You Healthy*. London: Atlantic.

Harrod Buhner, S. (2003). *The Fasting Path: The Way to Spiritual, Physical, and Emotional Enlightenment*. New York: Avery.

Hendel, B. & Ferreira, P. (2003). *Water & Salt: The Essence of Life*. Roseburg, OR: Natural Resources, Inc.

Huang, C. et al. (2002). Uric Acid and Urea in Human Sweat. *The Chinese Journal of Physiology*, 45(3): 109–115. Available at: https://www.researchgate.net/publication/10698087_Uric_acid_and_urea_in_human_sweat

Hobbs, C. (1992). *The Foundations of Health: A Liver and Digestive Herbal*. Capitola: Botanica Press.

Horton, R. (2020). COVID-19 is not a pandemic. *The Lancet*, 396(10255): 874.

Jackson, T. (2025). *The Care Economy*. Cambridge: Polity.

Jackson-Main, P. (2024). *The Mind's Eye: Personality and Behaviour as Revealed in Quantum Iris Analysis*. London: Aeon.

Jackson-Main, P. (2023). *Practical Iridology: Using the Eye as a Guide to Health Risks and Wellbeing*. London: Aeon.

Jarcho, S. (1970). Galen's Six Non-naturals: A Bibliographic Note and Translation. *Bulletin of the History of Medicine*, 44(4): 372–377. Available at: http://www.jstor.org/stable/44450783

Jensen, B. (2011). *Tissue Cleansing through Bowel Management*. Escondido: Bernard Jensen Enterprises.

Julian of Norwich. (2015). *Revelations of Divine Love*. Tr. Windeatt, B. Oxford: Oxford University Press.

Kaptchuk, T. (2000). *Chinese Medicine: The Web that has no Weaver*. London: Rider.

Kloss, J. (2004). *Back to Eden*. Silver Lake: Lotus Press.

Lachman, G. (2011). *The Quest for Hermes Trismegistus*. Edinburgh: Floris Books.

Lindlahr, H. (2014). *Nature Cure*. Independently Published.

Lipton, B. (2005). *The Biology of Belief: Unleashing the Power of Consciousness, Matter and Miracles*. Santa Rosa: Mountain of Love/Elite Books.
McKenna, P. (2007). *I Can Make You Thin*. London: Bantam Press.
Mendelsohn, R. (1990). *Confessions of a Medical Heretic*. New York: McGraw-Hill.
Milgrom, L. (2008). A New Geometrical Description of Entanglement and the Curative Homeopathic Process. *The Journal of Alternative and Complementary Medicine*, 14(3): 329–339.
Millman, O. (2022). *Can Geoengineering Fix the Climate? Hundreds of Scientists Say Not So Fast*. Available at: https://www.theguardian.com/environment/2022/dec/25/can-controversial-geoengineering-fix-climate-crisis
Moritz, A. (2012). *The Amazing Liver and Gallbladder Flush*. ebook: Ener-chi.com.
Muraki, I. et al. (2013). Fruit consumption and risk of type 2 diabetes: results from three prospective longitudinal cohort studies. *BMJ*, 347. doi: https://doi.org/10.1136/bmj.f5001
Ngan, A. & Conduit, R. (2011). A Double-blind, Placebo-controlled Investigation of the Effects of *Passiflora incarnata* (Passionflower) Herbal Tea on Subjective Sleep Quality. *Phytotherapy Research (PTR)*, 25(8): 1153–1159. doi: 10.1002/ptr.3400
Nunez, K. (2020). *What Is Shungite and Does It Have Healing Properties?* Available at: https://www.healthline.com/health/shungite
Ornish Lifestyle Medicine. (2023). *Empowering You*. Available at: https://learninggnm.com/documents/hamerbio.html
Pollan, M. (2008). In Defence of Food. *The Sunday Times*. Available at: https://www.thetimes.com/article/in-defence-of-food-by-michael-pollan-tvb5tft39v6?id=17515457033&medium=cpc&gad_source=5
Ristik, A. (2022). 15 Health Benefits of Sunlight + Dangers & Safety Tips. Available at: https://health.selfdecode.com/blog/avoiding-sun-will-kill-14-proven-science-based-health-benefits-sun/
Roth, G. (1990). *Maps to Ecstasy: Teachings of an Urban Shaman*. Wellingborough: Aquarian Press.
Schulze, R. (1995). *Cures from the Last-Chance Clinic: An Introduction to the Methods of an Herbal Master*. Charlottesville: The University of Natural Healing.
Selye, H. (1956). *The Stress of Life*. New York: McGraw-Hill.
Sharan, F. (1994). *Herbs of Grace: Becoming Independently Healthy*. Boulder: Wisdome Press.
Sharma, M. & Sharma, A. (2023). A Review on Nature Based Sunscreen Agents. *IOP Conference Series: Earth and Environmental Science*, Vol. 1110. Available at: https://iopscience.iop.org/article/10.1088/1755-1315/1110/1/012047

Sheldrake, M. (2023). *Entangled Life: How Fungi Make Our Worlds*. London: Bodley Head.

Stone, R. (1986). *Polarity Therapy*, Vols 1 & 2. Sebastopol, CA: CRCS Publications.

Szekely, E.B. (2018). *The Essene Gospel of Peace*. Audio Enlightenment Press.

Trebing, W.P. (2004). *Good-Bye Germ Theory: Ending a Century of Medical Fraud*. Bloomington: Xlibris.

UK Government (2024). *What is the WHO Pandemic Preparedness Treaty?* https://commonslibrary.parliament.uk/research-briefings/cbp-9550/

Want, A. (2019). A Brief History of Colour Vision. *Eye News*, 25(6). Available at: https://www.eyenews.uk.com/education/trainees/post/a-brief-history-of-colour-vision

Wardle, J., Steel, A., Lauche, R. & Adams, J. (2017). Collaborating with Medicine? Perceptions of Australian Naturopaths on Integrating within the Conventional Medical System. *Journal of Interprofessional Care*, 31(6): 734–743. Available at: http://www.tandfonline.com/doi/full/10.1080/13561820.2017.1351424

Watzeck, J.R. (2021). *Climate as a Weapon of War: H.A.A.R.P High Frequency Active Auroral Research Program*. Independently Published.

WHO. (2020). Coronavirus disease (COVID-19): Herd immunity, lockdowns and COVID-19. Available at: https://www.who.int/news-room/questions-and-answers/item/herd-immunity-lockdowns-and-covid-19

Willow, K. (2019). *German New Medicine Experiences in Practice: An Introduction to the Discoveries of Dr Ryke Geerd Hamer*. Independently Published.

Yancey, P. (1987). *Fearfully and Wonderfully Made*. Grand Rapids: Zondervan.

Young, Robert O. (2009). *The pH Miracle*. London: Piatkus.

INDEX

Note: References following "n" refer notes.

acid/alkaline food chart, 19
acute inflammation, 4
adaptogen, 45, 129, 130
adaptogenic plants, 105
Advil, 145
affirmations, 181–184
agni, 74
airborne threats, 98–101
aircraft trails, 98
Allen, W., 137
allostatic load, 7
all-purpose blend, 85
aloe species plants, 36
aluminium, 97
ama, 74
"amateur", 135
The Amazing Liver and Gallbladder Flush (Moritz), 170
ambient air, 93
    airborne threats and defences, 98–101
    aircraft trails, 98

aluminium, 97
atmospheric health risks, 94–98
cirrus homogenitus, 95
defensive strategies, 98–101
electromagnetic exposure, 103–106
electromagnetic soup, 103–106
geoengineering, 94–98
heavy metal detox, 102–103
post-vaccine symptom management, 102–103
sunlight and skin, 106–108
anorexigenic, 75
anthraquinone glycosides, 36
antioxidant, 82, 105, 107
antiporters, 22, 29
anxiety, endogenous, 116
art of doing nothing, 120–121
Asclepius, 1
ashwagandha (*Withania somnifera*), 105, 117

astragalus (*Astragalus membranaceous*), 101, 105
autoimmune conditions, 4–5
autointoxication, 22, 74
Avicenna, 163, 168, 179
awakening, 119–120

Bach, E., 130
Bach Flower Repertory, 130–131
Bach, R., 188
"Back to Nature", 67
barberry bark, 36, 37, 40
barley grain, 46
Batmanghelidj, F., 86
Béchamp, P. A., 18, 33n2
Bernard, C., 18
beta-glucuronidase, 22
The Birth of the Clinic (Foucault), 158
bitter tonics, 29
Blended Salad, 57, 85
blood-cleansing "alterative" herbs, 47
blue zones, 122–123
bodywork, 50, 133–134
Bone, K., 51
bowel cleanse, 35
    bowel motility capsules, 36–37
    coffee enema, 41–42
    colonics and enemas, 39–41
    diet, 39
    drawing powder, 37–39
    herbal formulae, 35
bowel health, 22–25
Boyd, D., 188
BPA (bisphenol A), 88
Brauchle, A., 187
breathing, deep, 50
Bristol Stool Chart, 25
Burroughs, S., 43

Campbell, P., 66
Cannon, W., 2, 13n5
The Care Economy (Jackson), 158
cascara sagrada bark, 36, 37
cayenne, 17, 30, 43, 44–45, 151, 153
Celtic sea salt, 88

central sensitization syndrome (CSS), 104
Champion juicer, 84
childbirth, natural, 151–154
chlorophyll, 82
cholecystitis, 46
Christopher, J.R., 1, 8, 10, 35, 37, 71, 74, 151, 163, 167, 168, 176, 178
chronic inflammation, 4
chronic kidney disease (CKD), 45
cirrus homogenitus, 95
Claudius Galenus. *See* Galen
cleavers, 51
clinical evidence, 162–163
coffee enema, 41–42
colonics, 39–41
colour-codes foods, 81–83
Confessions of a Medical Heretic (Mendelsohn), 162
conscious healing, 183–184
convalescence, 187
cooked food, 85–86
Cordyceps militaris, 46
core belief, 181
Covid-19, 23, 99
    EMF theory, 103
    herd immunity, 160–161
    post vaccine symptom management, 102–103
Cowan, T., 103
curcumin, 177, 178
Cures from the Last Chance Clinic (Schulze), 147
CYP3A4, 27
CYP450 isoenzyme supergene family, 27

D'Adamo, P., 66
Dahlke, R., 188
Damask rose, 129
dandelion (*Taraxacum officinale*), 40, 47
Dang Shen, 130
deep breathing, 50
defensive living, 87–89
Deruelle, F., 98, 108n9
Descartes, R., 92n18

detox diary, sample, 62–63
detoxification, 12, 15, 83, 99
    acid/alkaline food chart, 19
    antiporters, 29
    bitter tonics, 29
    bowel cleanse, 35–42
    bowel health, 22–25
    Bristol Stool Chart, 25
    chart of iris topography, 23, 24
    detox tea, 47–49
    "evacuation of superfluities", 20
    experience over theory, 15–17
    food intake, 56–57
    5-day "fast-track" detox, 59–61
    gastrocolic reflex, 25
    Germ theory, 17–18
    heavy metal detox, 102–103
    homeostasis, 18
    indications for, 32
    inflammation, 18
    juicing for detox, 83–85
    key organs in, 21–31
    kidneys, 25–26, 42–46
    liver, 22, 26–29, 46–49
    lungs, 31, 56
    lymphatic system, 29–30, 50–51
    metabolism, 20
    one-month detox programme, 58
    practical, 35
    sample detox diary, 62–63
    seasonal and situational detox, 57–58
    simplest routine, 17
    skin, 30–31, 52–56
    stagnation, 20, 31
    Terrain Theory, 17–21
    terrain-modulation, 21
    tissue encumbrance, 20–21
    xenotoxins, 27
Diamond, H., 66, 74, 78
Diamond, M., 66, 74, 78
diaphoretics, 30
diet, 49, 51
    bowel cleanse, 39
    contemporary, 28

Hay Diet, 77
health-supporting, 28
optimising, 16, 27
plant-based, 79
vegetarian, 68–69, 80
digestion, 21, 74–76, 82
    bitter tonics, 29
    food combining, 77–79
    food energetics, 85–86
    mindful eating, 76–77
    overeating, 74
digoxin, 142
distillation, 88
doctor, 167
drawing powder, 37–39
dreaming, 118–119
dry skin brushing, 50, 52–53
dysbiosis, 24

eating
    meat-eating, 80, 81
    mindful eating, 76–77
    overeating, 74
    personalised approaches, 65–67
Eat Right 4 Your Type (D'Adamo), 66
Eat Right, Lose Weight (Campbell), 66
echinacea (*Echinacea angustifolia, E. purpurea*), 51, 100, 164
Edison, T., 178
Ehret, A., 37, 74
elecampane (*Inula helenium*), 100
electromagnetic exposure, 103–106
electromagnetic frequencies (EMFs), 93
    specific toxicity, 105
    theory, 103
electromagnetic soup, 103–106
emergency medicine, 145–151
"endogenous" anxiety, 116
enemas, 39–41
entanglement, 3
The Essene Gospel of Peace (Szekely), 1, 13n2
"evacuation of superfluities", 20
exercise, 30, 50, 111–114, 120–121, 122, 123, 185

fasting, 90–91
The Fasting Path (Buhner), 91
Fennell, J., 111
filtration, 88
Fit for Life (H. and M. Diamond), 66
5-day "fast-track" detox, 59–61
"5-Rhythms", 132
Flexner, A., 1
food, 67
    acid/alkaline food chart, 19
    colour-codes, 81–83
    combining, 77–79
    cooked food, 85–86
    energetics, 85–86
    intake, 56–57
    nutrition in synthetic age, 71–74
    processing, 70–71
    raw food, 85–86
    sample food diary, 89
    Schulze's Superfood, 57
    supplements, 71–74, 91n2
    3Ps, 70, 86
    wholefood movement, 67
    whole foods to processed diets, 67–71
"forever chemicals", 21
Foucault, M., 158
The Foundations of Health (Hobbs), 74
fruit, 28, 43, 78, 85, 92n8
fullerenes, 105–106

Galen, 6, 13n8
gastrocolic reflex, 25
Gates, B., 94
geoengineering, 96
Germ theory, 17–18
ghrelin, 75
gut-associated lymphatic tissues (GALT), 23

HAARP (High-frequency Active Auroral Research Program), 96
haemoglobin, 82
Hamer, R. G., 131–132
Harrod Buhner, S., 91
Hay Diet, 77
Hay, W. H., 77

healing, 188. *See also* natural healing
    conscious, 183–184
    energy, 3
    myths of, 10
    politics, 158, 164
    self-determined, 168–169
    state, 184–187
    time, 187–188
    within, 188–189
    inner voice of, 181–184
The Healing Power of Illness (Thorwald & Dahlke), 2, 188
healing space, 175, 184
    affirmations, 181–184
    conscious healing, 183–184
    cultivating mindset for recovery, 175–176
    healing state, 184–187
    healing within, 188–189
    health beliefs, 176–180
    innate healing power, 180–181
    inner voice of healing, 181–184
    time to heal, 187–188
health autonomy, 166
    incurable people, 168–169
    living and dying, 169–170
    self-determined healing, 168–169
    suppression of, 163
health beliefs, 176–180
healthcare freedom, 158
    clinical evidence, 162–163
    herd immunity, 160–161
    immunity illusion, 161–162
    informed consent, 159
    integrated medicine, 164–166
    medical self-empowerment, 164–166
    political struggle of natural medicine, 164
    politics of healing, 158
    suppression of healing autonomy, 163
    vaccine narrative, 160
    whoops factor in medicine, 162
health-enhancing practices, 105
heavy metal detox, 102–103
herbal tea recipe, 118

Herb Doc, 134, 148
herd immunity, 160–161
Hermes Trismegistus, 1
Himalayan crystal salt, 88
"hippie" movement, 67
Hobbs, C., 74
homeostasis, 18
hormesis, 121–123
Horsetail herb (*Equisetum arvense*), 103
Horton, R., 161
hydration, 86–87
hydrotherapy, 50, 53–54
Hygieia, 1
hyperbaric oxygen tents, 100
hypnotic herbs, 116–117

"iatrogenic", 141
iatrogenic illness, 141–145
Ibn Bhutlan, 20
Ice Man. *See* Wim Hof
immunity illusion, 161–162
incurable people, 168–169
inflammation, 4, 18
informed consent, 159
innate healing power, 180–181
    affirmations, 181–184
    conscious healing, 183–184
    healing state, 184–187
    inner voice of healing, 181–184
inner voice of healing, 181–184
insomnia, 115
integrated medicine, 164–166
intermittent fasting, 90
"intestinal broom", 37
Intestinal Formulae (IF), 36–37
iris topography chart, 23, 24
Iyengar, B. K. S., 114

Jackson, T., 158
Jensen, B., 23, 37, 41, 53
juicing, 83–85

Kaqun water, 100, 108n10
kidney, 25–26
    flush, 42–46
    kidney-bladder tea, 45
Koch, R., 17

lemons, 43, 85
leptin, 75
"life energy", 20
lifestyle balance, 109
    blue zones, 122–123
    exercise, 111
    hormesis, 121–123
    moving your body, 111–114
    personalising health, 109–111
    sleep, 114–120
    subtle art of doing nothing, 120–121
    "walking the dog", 111–112
limes, 43, 85
liver, 22, 26–29
    detoxification, 99
    flush, 46–49
    "Polarity Liver Flush", 46
    stagnation, 28
living, defensive, 87–89
local grassroots initiatives, 73
Long Covid, 99
Love Your Disease, It's Keeping You Healthy (Harrison), 2
lungs, 31, 56, 100–101
lymph, 29
lymphatic system, 23, 29–30
    bodywork, 50
    deep breathing, 50
    diet, 51
    dry skin brushing, 50
    exercise, 50
    herbs, 51
    hydrotherapy, 50
lymph nodes, 29
lymph system. *See* lymphatic system

macrophages, 29, 51
manual lymphatic drainage (MLD), 50
marshmallow (*Althaea officinalis*), 40, 101
"Master Cleanser" routine, 43
masticating juicers, 84
McKenna, P., 76
Mead, M., 146

meat-eating, 80, 81
medical self-empowerment, 164–166
Mendelsohn, R.S., 162
metabolism, 20, 65–67
mind and body interconnectedness,
    125–128
mindful eating, 76–77
The Mind's Eye (Jackson-Main), 3, 119,
    127, 134, 159, 180
mood-enhancers, 129
    codonopsis (*Codonopsis pilosula*),
        129–130
    lemon balm (*Melissa officinalis*), 129
    rose (*Rosa damascena*), 129
    rosemary (*Rosmarinus officinalis*),
        130
    Siberian ginseng (*Eleutherococcus
        senticosus*), 129
Moritz, A., 46, 170
mucilaginous herbs, 40
mullein (*Verbascum thapsus*), 100

natural healing, 1, 139. *See also*
        healing
    case studies, 141–154
    childbirth, 151–154
    cleansing and rebuilding, 12
    commitment to change, 11
    emergency medicine, 145–151
    finding healing path, 140–141
    great myths of healing, 10
    healing power of nature, 2–6
    iatrogenic illness, 141–145
    limits and integration of,
        139–140
    Natural Healing Filter, 7–10
    natural history of inflammation, 4
    personal journey, 157
    pillars of, 12
    responsibility, 11
    simplicity, 11
    Six Non-Naturals, 6–7
    "Unity of Disease", 11
Natural Healing Filter, 7
nature cure. *See* natural healing
naturopathy. *See* natural healing

nettle, 45
neurogenic iris types, 186
neurogenics, 186
Newton, I., 183
Nietzsche, F., 122
non-local effects, 3
nourishment, 65
    digestion, 74–79
    fasting, 90–91
    food, 67–74
    nutrition in synthetic age, 71–74
    personalised approaches, 65–67
    phytonutrients, 82
    plant-based paradox, 79–81
    plant colours and nutrients, 81–86
    sample food diary, 89
    water, 86–89

objectivist paradigm, 179
one-month detox programme, 58
Operating Department Assistant
        (ODA), 150
Ornish, D., 144
overeating, 74
oxidative stress, 104
oxytocin, 134

parasympathetic nervous system
        (PSNS), 115
passionflower (*Passiflora incarnata*), 117
Pasteur, L., 17
personal health plan check list, 172
personalising health, 109–111
"pharmocentric society", 143
pH Miracle recipe, 57
physical movement, 131–132
phytonutrients, 82
plantain (*Plantago lanceolata, P. major*), 101
plant
    -based, 79–81
    essences, 130
    medicine, 128–130
plant nutrients, 81
    colour-codes foods, 81–83
    cooked vs. raw food, 85–86
    juicing, 83–85

pleural effusion, 142
pneuma, 3, 20
"Polarity Liver Flush", 46
Polarity Therapy, 46, 50
polio vaccine, 173n7
Pollan, M., 67, 74, 79, 80
post-vaccine symptom management, 102–103
Practical Iridology (Jackson-Main), 17, 19, 114, 189n1
prana, 3, 20
pranayama, 3
processing, 70–71
psychiatric illness, 132
pungent herbs, 30, 36

qi, 3, 20, 92n13
qi tonic, 101

raw food, 85–86
relationships, 136–137
respiratory herbs, 100–101
rest, 114–117. *See also* sleep
Rhodiola, 129
Roth, G., 132

St John's wort (*Hypericum perforatum*), 128
Salk vaccine, 173n7
Schulze, R., 7, 8, 10, 31, 35, 46, 145, 146, 147
Schulze's Superfood, 57
seasonal affective disorder (SAD syndrome), 107
seasonal and situational detox, 57
self-determined healing, 168–169
Selye, H., 13n5, 119
senna, 36
17-Herb detox tea, 48
Shen tonic, 128
shungite, 105
Siberian ginseng (*Eleutherococcus senticosus*), 105
situational detox, 57
skin, 30–31, 52
    clothes and topical products, 55–56

dry skin brushing, 52–53
hydrotherapy, 53–54
and sunlight, 106–108
topical treatments, 55
sleep, 114, 115
    awakening, 119–120
    dreaming, 118–119
    herbal tea recipe, 118
    rest through Chinese medicine, 114–117
    sleep hygiene, 117–118
    traditional Chinese medicine organ clock, 116
space of healing. *See* healing space
Special Detox tea, 102
spleen, 92n13
spleen qi deficiency, 85
stagnation, 20, 31
standard medicine, 159
Stephenson, R., 179
stimulating herbs, 36
Stone, R., 46
stratospheric aerosol injection (SAI), 98
stress, 125
    Bach Flower Repertory, 130–131
    bodywork, 133–134
    healing through movement, 131–132
    interconnectedness of mind and body, 125–128
    passion and path, 134–136
    physical movement, 131–132
    plant essences, 130
    plant medicine, 128–130
    relationships, 136–137
    "5-Rhythms", 132
    Shen tonic, 128
    St John's wort (*Hypericum perforatum*), 128
    "stress-related" illness, 127
    thymoleptics, 129
The Stress of Life (Selye), 13n5
sunlight, 106–108
supplements, 71–74, 91n2
sympathetic nervous system (SNS), 115
Szekely, E.B., 1

tea
    detox tea, 47–49
    herbal tea recipe, 118
    17-Herb detox tea, 48
    kidney-bladder tea, 45
    Special Detox tea, 102
terrain-modulation, 21
Terrain Theory, 17–21
thoracic duct, 50
Thorwald, D., 188
Thoth. *See* Hermes Trismegistus
3Ps, 70, 86
thyme (*Thymus officinalis*), 101
thymoleptics, 129
Tissue Cleansing through Bowel Management (Jensen), 37
tissue encumbrance, 20–21
topical treatments, 55
traditional Chinese medicine organ clock, 116
traditional medicine diagnostic techniques, 20
trauma healer, 128

"Unity of Disease", 11

vaccine narrative, 160
Virchow, R., 18
Vital Force, 175
Vogel, A., 180

"walking the dog", 111–112
Warburg, O., 18
warming spices, 47
water, 86
    defensive living, 87–89
    distillation, 88
    filtration, 88
    hydration, 86–87
wellness spectrum, 157
    health autonomy, 166–167
    healthcare freedom, 158–164
    navigating, 170–172
    patient to practitioner, 166–167
    personal health plan check list, 172
white carbs, 51
wholefood movement, 67
whoops factor in medicine, 162
Wim Hof, 54
The Wisdom of the Body (Cannon), 2, 13n5

xenotoxins, 27

yang, 114
yellow dock root, 39–40
yin, 114
Young, E., 186
Young, Robert O., 57, 78, 92n8

www.ingramcontent.com/pod-product-compliance
Ingram Content Group UK Ltd.
Pitfield, Milton Keynes, MK11 3LW, UK
UKHW050825040126
466577UK00004B/23